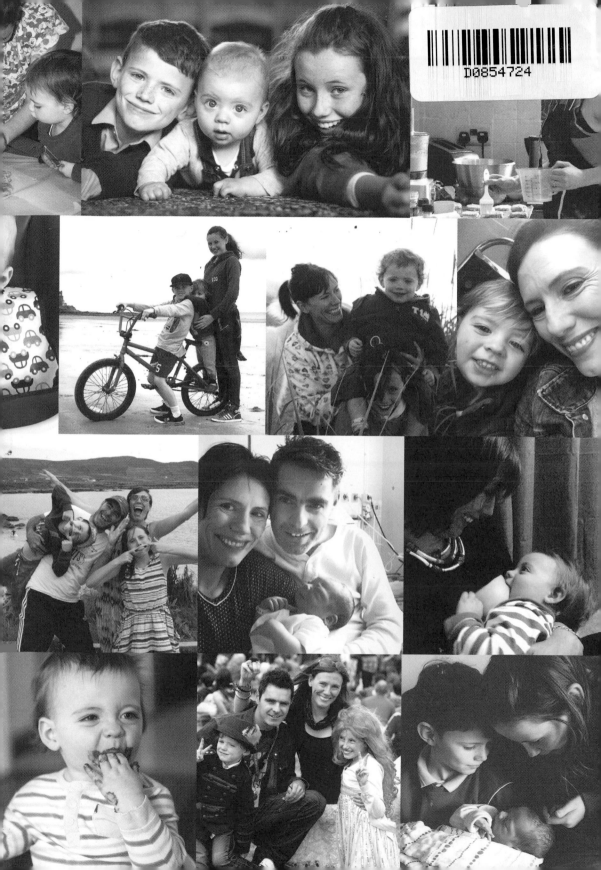

THE
BABY-LED FEEDING
COOKBOOK

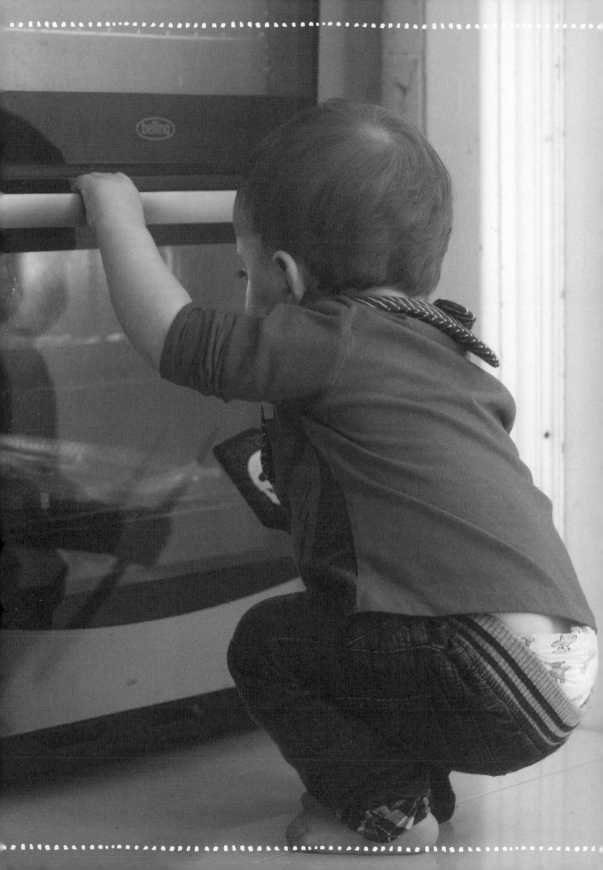

THE
BABY-LED FEEDING
COOKBOOK

A new healthy way of eating for your
baby that the whole family will love!

AILEEN COX BLUNDELL

GILL BOOKS

Gill Books
Hume Avenue
Park West
Dublin 12
www.gillbooks.ie

Gill Books is an imprint of M.H. Gill & Co.

© Aileen Cox Blundell 2017

978 07171 7263 4

Photography and food styling by Aileen Cox Blundell
Designed by Aileen Cox Blundell
Illustrations by Niamh Harman
Edited by Emma Dunne
Indexed by Eileen O'Neill
Printed by BZ Graf, Poland

This book is typeset in 9.5pt on 12.5pt Chaparral Pro.

The paper used in this book comes from the wood pulp of
managed forests. For every tree felled, at least one tree is
planted, thereby renewing natural resources.

A CIP catalogue record for this book is available from the
British Library.

5 4 3 2 1

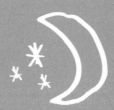

For my beautiful children, Jade, Dylan and Oscar.
Thank you all so much for picking me to be your
momma. It's the best privilege in the world and
I love you all to the moon and back.

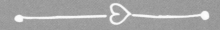

Note

Information given in this book is not intended to be taken as a replacement for medical advice. Always consult a qualified medical practitioner before introducing food to your baby.

The Author

Aileen Cox Blundell grew up in a little village in Westmeath. She loved to help her mother cook, and it was there, at home, that she developed her passion for healthy, wholesome food.

When her daughter Jade was born in 2002, the only way to get her to eat anything was to place the food in front of her and let her take control and feed herself. Seeing the incredible benefits of allowing her children to experiment with food at an early age led her to create the blog and website Baby-Led Feeding. When she isn't cooking or developing exciting new recipes, Aileen runs a successful design studio specialising in branding and packaging for various food companies. She lives in Swords with her husband, Conor, and their three foodie children, Jade, Dylan and Oscar.

Acknowledgements

First, to all the mums and dads out there who have been such a tremendous part of the baby-led feeding community from the start: you are all amazing and I love that you try so hard to encourage your little ones to love good food. It's not an easy task and it takes work and commitment but you are making a huge difference to their future health.

To the love of my life, Conor: thank you for your encouragement, support and patience and, most importantly, for teaching me how to use the camera properly. Sorry for being a terrible student at times. You did so much extra work around the house so I could write a book and I love you for it. You're my rock and the best dad in the world to our three children.

To all the people at Gill Books, especially Catherine Gough and Emma Lynam: thank you for believing I could do this and for the opportunity to write this book. You have given me so much encouragement and I'm so proud to have signed with you. To Roisin Gowan: thank you so much for your support and for contributing a foreword to this book.

To my mam: thank you so much for being the best mam in the world, for teaching me how to cook and for giving me a love of food. To my dad: thank you for the fish, the pheasant and the craic. You're my number-one fan and I'm yours. I've always been proud of how hard you worked to provide for us. To my other mammy, Annette: thank you for tasting so much food and for your admirable honesty. You're the best nana ever!

To Christopher, Sheena, Darren, Ciara, Gillian, Orla, Daire, Laura, all my friends called Sarah, Clair, Niamh and Jenna: thank you for everything! For tasting, for the encouragement, for the honest critique of the food and for still being my friends even after not seeing me for months on end. I love you all.

To baby Addison and baby Jody: thank you for being my little taste testers. I love being your godmother.

And last but not least, to my friend Natasha: I'm sure you didn't expect to see your name here but without you this book would not be possible. You're so inspiring and I love that you believed in me. It meant the world to me.

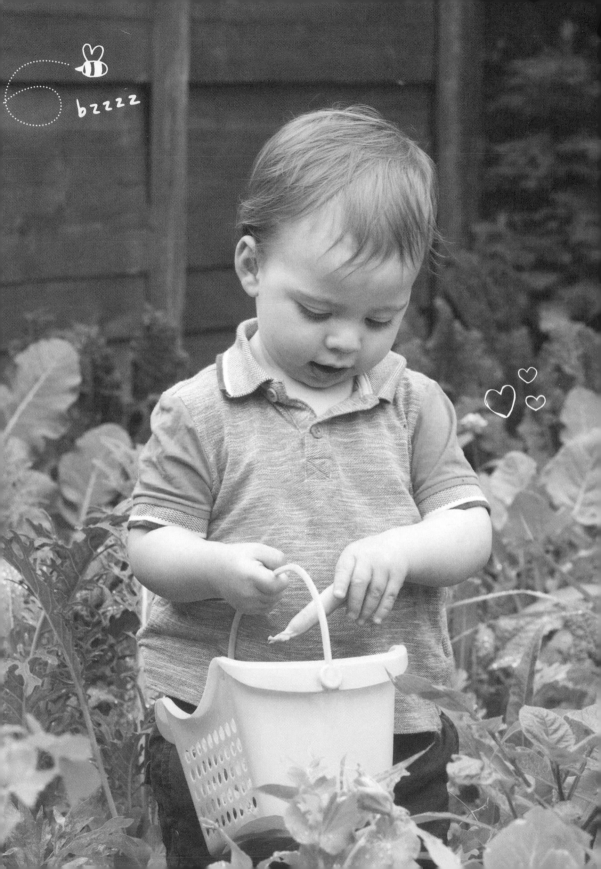

Foreword

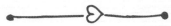

As a paediatric dietitian, I am dedicated to helping parents make healthy choices for their little ones. From the moment I met Aileen, I was impressed by her passion, enthusiasm and common-sense approach to creating recipes for baby-led feeding.

Baby-led feeding is an exciting way to expose your child to a variety of tastes and textures from the start of their lives, and it can also make mealtimes more fun. It can help improve hand–eye coordination and the development of healthy eating habits as children learn to self-regulate their feeding. Babies can independently pace their eating, satisfy their appetites and meet their individual nutritional requirements. This book is designed with that in mind.

It also provides healthy choices for your little ones. Aileen has created delicious meals and natural treats with less than the recommended sugar intake for each serving. Limiting this type of sugar can reduce the risk of health problems such as childhood obesity and type 2 diabetes.

This book is the product of a lot of hard work, dedication and determination. It is a fantastic guide to teaching your baby to enjoy a variety of tasty foods and drinks, and I would be happy to recommend it to my clients!

I hope you enjoy this book as much as I did.

Roisin Gowan,
Registered Senior Paediatric Dietitian,
works in Ireland's biggest children's hospital, is
registered with CORU and is a member of the INDI

Contents

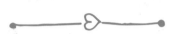

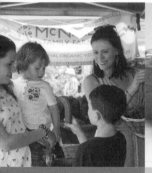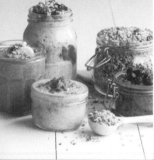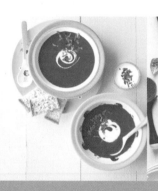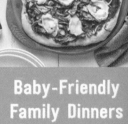

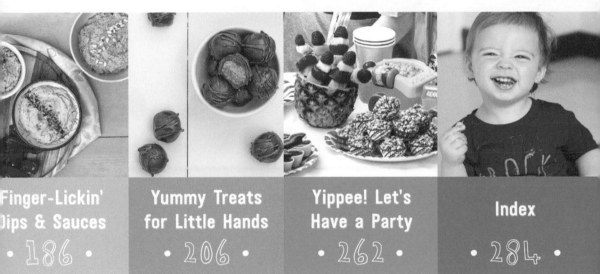

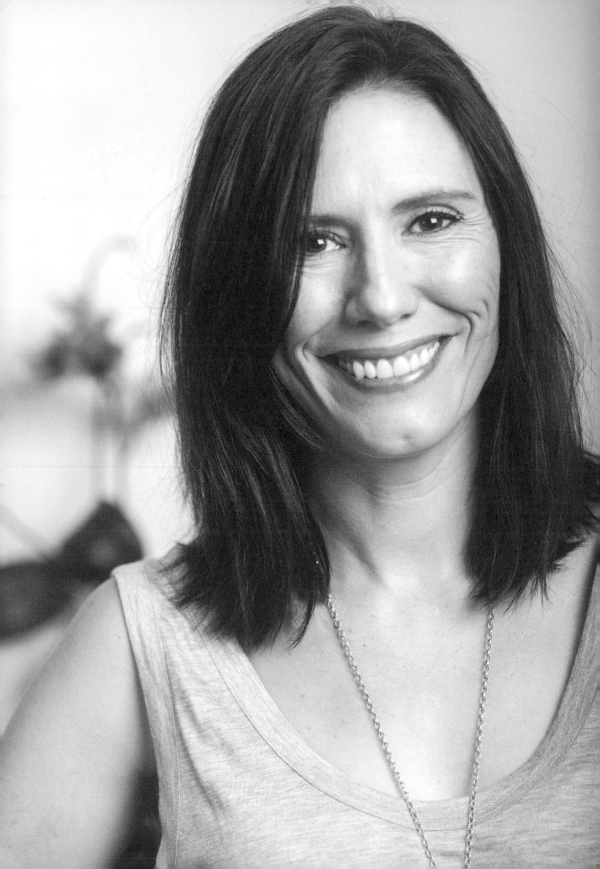

Introduction
my story

Ever since I was a little girl, I have always had a passion for food, both cooking and eating it. I can vividly remember running home from school to help my mother bake bread or prepare stew for dinner. I think she instinctively knew that getting kids involved in cooking made their love of food even stronger.

I grew up in a little village in Westmeath called Multyfarnham. Imagine lush green fields, farm after farm and lots and lots of lakes. My dad taught me how to fish and each season we would fill the freezer up to the brim with fresh trout and salmon. In the winter months, when the fishing season was over, he hunted for wild pheasant and duck and these were our staple meats for most of my childhood.

As a child, though, I thought we must be very poor to be eating like this and, like most kids, I wanted the things I couldn't have – white bread, chocolate breakfast cereals and anything besides trout or pheasant for dinner.

In my teenage years, I worked in kitchens as a trainee chef. The hours were long, the work was hard and it just didn't seem like a job that would make me truly happy in the end. I decided that it wasn't the life for me and that I would rather keep my love of cooking at home for myself and my friends and family, and instead I pursued a career in graphic design.

My daughter Jade was born in San Francisco when I was twenty-five years old and right from the moment she entered my life I naturally wanted only the best for her. I breastfed her exclusively until she started solids and then began introducing a varied diet of fish, meats, vegetables and fruits – all puréed into the craziest of concoctions. Everything was going great until Jade reached seven months old and decided she no longer wanted me to feed her with a spoon. She would simply turn her head to the side, purse her lips and refuse point blank to let me put any food into her mouth. The only way I could get her to eat anything was to place the food in front of her and let her take control and feed herself.

I was a first-time momma. I was anxious and worried whether she was getting enough food, let alone the nutrients she needed to grow healthy and strong. Baby-led feeding wasn't even a phrase yet – and wouldn't be till almost six years later. I didn't know anyone who had experienced this with their baby and no one had any advice to give me. So I brought her to my paediatrician – she saw the panic-stricken look on my face and instantly put her hand on my shoulder and told me I was to trust my instincts as a mother. She said to remember that milk comes first and that once I gave her healthy, nutritious foods Jade would be fine.

Over the following years Jade showed me how capable she was at demolishing every food I put in front of her. Nothing was off the menu and by the time she was three years old she ate everything from sushi to olives and spicy chicken. It was amazing to all those around us how much of a little foodie she had become.

My son Dylan was born five years later and was a whopping almost-eleven-pound baby boy who just loved food! When it came to weaning, I'm not sure why I didn't adopt the method I had ended up using with Jade, but again I decided to opt for the more traditional method with him. It seemed like the easiest thing to purée all of his meals and, at the beginning, once there was food he didn't care how it arrived – until he got his toddler independence.

There was a lot of 'here comes the train' and 'quick before Daddy eats your dinner', but no amount of pleading would get my two-year-old to eat. In restaurants, my husband and I took it in turns to spoon food into him while the other ate their dinner, so one of us always ate cold food.

As Dylan got older, broccoli became trees, asparagus became giraffe's legs and spinach was superhero food – all superheros eat spinach! Believe me, when your kid is fussy you'll do anything to try get them to like more things. Dinners were stressful, trying to get him to eat the meals we had made, and in the end we created the 'list of five things'. He could pick five things he didn't like and we wouldn't put them on his plate. But he was such a clever little thing that he would ask before dinner what we were cooking and the list would change accordingly. So we had to change tactics. Our new solution was to get him to just try everything that was on his plate. One bite. Just one!

To grown-ups this seems really reasonable, but to a young child trying new things is daunting. What if they don't like it? It looks terrible so it probably tastes like it looks. The breakthrough came one day when we cut up a fresh, ready-to-eat ripe mango. My husband looked at him and asked him to have just a little taste, and he shook his head and said no. It took fifteen minutes of persuasion and tears until, finally, he put half a teaspoon into his mouth. His face suddenly changed from the 'I've just eaten a lemon' expression to joy and he said, 'I think my new favourite food is mango!'

This was just what we needed because in the years that followed we were able to use the mango story as leverage to get him to try new foods. He is still the pickiest eater of my three children but usually only about meat and fish these days. I have to give him huge credit for being such a great trier. He may not like everything but he tries and we are happy with that.

My own attitude to food has changed so much over the past ten years. In 2010 I took up running in an aim to get fit and healthy. I didn't do crazy amounts, just three or four runs a week, but instead of feeling the benefits of getting more exercise I felt worse. I was tired all the time, cranky, constantly getting sick and always feeling run down. I went to the doctor and had some blood tests but nothing seemed to be out of the ordinary. I just seemed to be constantly trying to make myself feel like I had the energy to get through the day. Most days I had chocolate and Coke and that helped – for about an hour; then I went back to feeling like rubbish.

I did eat lots of vegetables and fruit, but it wasn't until I decided that something had to give and started writing down the foods I ate that I realised how much bad food I was putting into my body. It wasn't just weekend treats, which is what I had convinced myself I was having: it had become a daily thing.

It just so happened that around this time there seemed to be documentary after documentary on TV on the effects of processed foods and sugar. And it dawned on me, finally, how food really has such an effect on our well-being. There is something so powerful when you understand what food does to your body.

So that was my wake-up call, and I took control of my own health. Back to the basics I went -- to fresh, whole foods, natural produce and, most importantly, packaging free (which is also better for the environment). I cooked everything from scratch and prepared wholesome treats made from ingredients I could pronounce. Within a few weeks, my skin had cleared, I slept well and I felt a million times better than I had ever done. I also noticed a huge difference in my children. They ate less sweet foods and way more vegetables, and treats became just what they should be: occasional – much to their dismay at times.

In 2013 I got pregnant with my beautiful Oscar and I felt so empowered by my newfound love of healthy foods that I wanted to pass this love to him. I also wanted to let him feed himself the way Jade had and so I started taking photos of his food adventures. Each week I would photograph him and catalogue the recipes I cooked for him. He was amazing to watch as he shoved pasta with beetroot pesto into his mouth, and baby pizzas and healthy kale muffins. I never gave him alternatives – if he didn't eat it the first time, I put it back in the fridge and gave it to him when he was hungry and it really worked.

the **family**

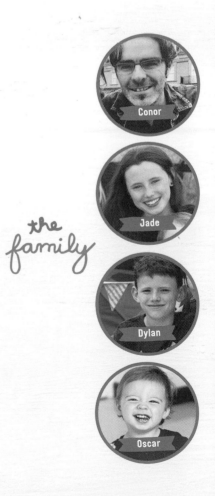

Conor

Jade

Dylan

Oscar

When Oscar was one I showed my lovely mother my collection of photos and recipes and, being the supportive mother she is, she encouraged me not hide them from the world but to use them to help other parents to get their babies to eat in a healthier way, and so the Baby-Led Feeding website was born.

I am overwhelmed by the response from the community of mothers and fathers who follow my blog and cook the food. Every day, families share their stories, make the foods from my recipes and, even better, send me cute photos of their children eating them. It encourages me so much to continue on this journey and to help make life easier for parents. There is enough to do without being tied to the cooker, and I hope this book shows you how easy it is to make healthy, nourishing food for your little ones.

All the recipes are made with your babies in mind. They are refined-sugar free, salt free and use as much fresh fruit and vegetables as I could possibly cram in. I'm really looking forward to your babies growing up with Baby-Led Feeding and I'm really excited to see what you all make.

Aileen xoxo

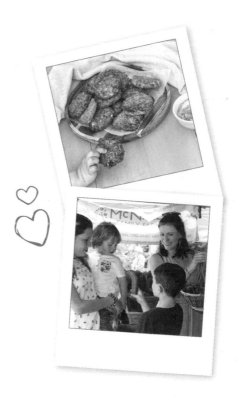

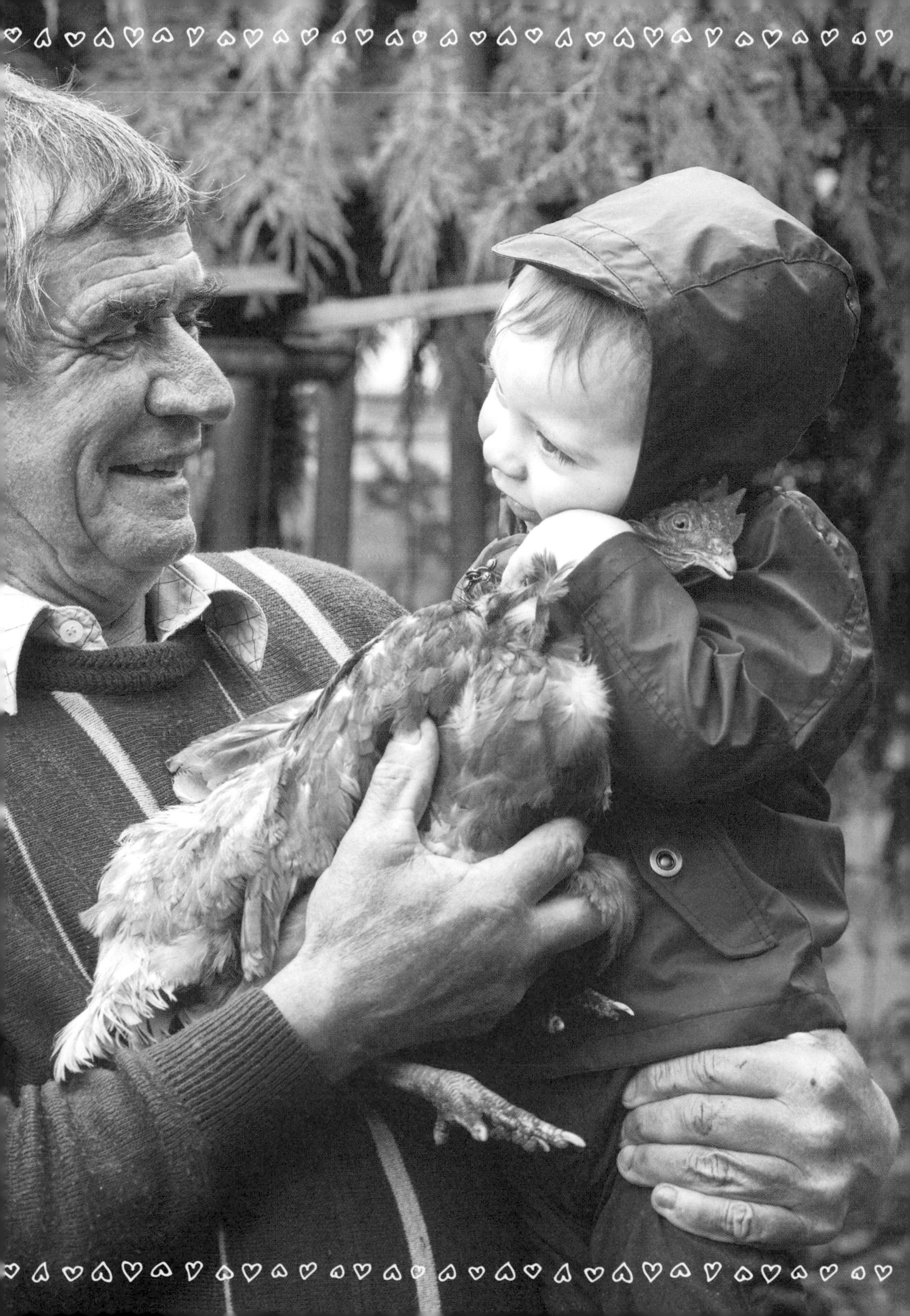

What Is
Baby-Led Feeding?

Baby-led feeding works from the same principles as baby-led weaning. It begins when your little one is around the six-month mark and has started to show signs of being able to pick up food.

You will know when your baby is ready when the piece of toast in your hand is suddenly being stuffed into their little mouth or your stem of broccoli disappears with only remnants left on your little baby's face.

It is this curiosity and adventure that makes baby-led feeding so special. It's a natural exploration of everything around them and this is encouraged by giving them wholesome and naturally delicious foods that they will grab, explore and put into their mouths all by themselves.

It is such an enjoyable time for the baby and the entire family. You get to watch this little human being you have brought into the world take complete control over what they eat. You watch them poke holes in muffins, peering in to see what the soft textures contain, and experience that joy of seeing them try a mushroom for the first time and loving it or hating it but knowing they picked up that food all by themselves, put it in their mouth and tried.

The main belief behind baby-led feeding is that all food should be healthy food, and with the growing statistics of obesity in Ireland, it is more important now than ever to make sure we are giving our children the right foods to help nourish them for the long term.

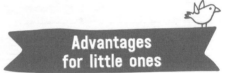

Advantages for little ones

1 Healthy food choice

If you only give your baby healthy food then that is what they will grow up knowing – good food is healthy food. It takes a while for your baby to happily munch on a lettuce leaf but you will be astounded when they do so for the first time.

2 Good eating habits – self-regulation

There are no spoons, no choo-choo trains, no 'Daddy's gonna eat your dinner'. Your baby gets to choose from here on in. They decide what they want to eat and what they don't, how much to eat and, more importantly, when they are full. I'm sure we all remember at some stage being told 'You're finished your dinner when your plate is empty'? Well, that all goes out the door from here on in.

Learning to chew first and then swallow

If a food is soft enough to squish between your finger and thumb then your baby's gums, even without teeth, are strong enough to break it down. This chewing develops naturally with the new foods you give your little one and also aids in the natural digestion of food.

 ### Learning about different textures and dexterity

Your baby will learn to explore and manage different textures and shapes of food from six months old. They will have the opportunity to practise their fine motor skills by grasping and picking up food at every meal.

 ### More likely to be better eaters

As your baby tries new foods, they will experience a world of new textures they would probably not have had the opportunity to try if they were traditionally weaned. This is so important because, in the long term, they will be more inclined to pick up and try new foods than 'taste with their eyes'. Babies who feed themselves are much less likely to be picky eaters – they want to see what this strange new food is that has been placed in front of them. Because your baby has been exposed to a variety of fresh and wholesome foods from the very beginning, they are much more likely to try a little taste of something new.

  ## Advantages for parents

 ### Less time-consuming

Your baby eats what you eat. There is no mashing concoctions of foods you probably wouldn't eat yourself: you simply cook healthy, delicious food for your family and then let your baby get to work on it on their own.

 ### Eating a warm dinner

The biggest plus for me is being able to eat my own dinner while my little one munches away on his own food. Because I'm not trying to get him to eat one more bite and he is eating at his own pace, we get to eat dinner as a family and it is so much more fun. Watching a seven-month-old feed himself spaghetti and meatballs while the rest of the family eats them too is what it's all about.

 ### Having a less-picky eater

This is a benefit not only for the child but also for the parents. It means you don't have to try and think of foods to give your baby while you cook something totally different for the rest of the family. We all eat the same and there are no alternatives.

Knowing you have a good eater on your hands

Many a person has been astounded over the past few years as my child demolishes an entire baby bowl of beetroot pasta. There is so much pleasure in knowing your child loves good food and will at least try everything you put in front of him.

Getting Started

So your baby has reached six months and is ready to eat solid foods. This is the most exciting time, as you get to watch them explore new textures, tastes and smells.

The great thing about the baby-led way of feeding is that you don't need much to get started, and even though you might be a bit skeptical that your six-month-old baby will be able to hold and eat an entire spear of avocado, they will amaze you with their talents. There are a few basic principles to follow when starting your baby-led journey.

Invest in a good high chair

I use a great one that straps to a normal chair. It was cheap and came with its own tray but can also be used without it, which means the baby can eat at the kitchen table with the rest of the family.

Buy a long-sleeved bib

There are many types of long-sleeved bibs out there and they are brilliant. They save on changing clothes after every meal and if you can get one with a catch pocket that's even better, as it reduces spillages on the floor.

Be prepared for a little bit of mess

At the same time, food mess from a little baby is fairly easy to clean up, and if your baby has a good plastic bib on then they shouldn't get that messy. Also, they become really good at eating really quickly. You just have to relax and go with it.

Invest in a wipeable tablecloth

Cut a wipeable tablecloth into quarters and place one clean piece under your baby's high chair. Any food that falls off can then be picked up and given back to them, which minimises any wastage.

Forget the bowl

Unless you can find a really good suction bowl your baby is just going to fling it across your kitchen floor. So just place the food onto their high-chair tray and let them get to work.

Teach them how to use cutlery

I gave my baby a kiddie spoon when he was about seven months old. At the start, he placed the food onto the spoon with one hand; then usually as he placed the spoon into his mouth the food fell off. But he learnt very quickly and by the time he was ten months old he was able to feed himself soup without spilling a drop ... well, most of the time.

Sometimes you have to pre-load a spoon

It is a messy affair watching your baby spoon-feed or fist-feed chia pudding into their mouth, so initially you may need to pre-load a spoon to help them on their way. This simply means you put the food on the spoon and let your baby pick it up and put it in their own mouth. Essentially, you are still not feeding them – they are doing the work. It's a great way for them to master the art of using cutlery, and before you know it they'll be drinking soup from a spoon on their own like a pro!

Let them use their hands

They will want to use their hands regardless of how messy the food is and will learn about so many textures and tastes.

Start slow

Introduce soft foods at the beginning like banana or roasted sweet potato. I also gave my kiddies roasted butternut squash, avocado, steamed carrots, broccoli and scrambled egg. It's so much fun watching them explore their new food and having that first magical taste.

Make it manageable

When you are giving fruits and vegetables on the side, cut them into thick chip sizes. This makes it much easier for small babies to manage, as they get frustrated if the food is too small to pick up. Just remember that all food should break apart when squashed between your thumb and index finger.

Ensure a balanced diet

Until babies are six months old, they get all the nutrition they need from either breastmilk or formula. After that, iron-rich and nutritious foods need to be introduced to their diet. According to Bord Bia: 'The best way to ensure that your child is eating a balanced diet is to offer a wide range of different foods each day.'

Rainbow of foods

Don't let them get to the angry hungry stage

Babies get frustrated when they are hungry so space out the milk feeds and solid-food feeds. Believe me, it makes for way more enjoyable meal times for everyone!

Eat together

It is lovely to eat as a family anyway, but when it comes to letting babies feed themselves, it's even better. You don't have to disrupt your own meal by trying to get them to eat. And seeing everyone eating the same foods will encourage your baby to try them too. You simply all eat together and I guarantee that seeing your little one feed themselves will bring a whole new joy to your mealtimes.

Enjoy it

Baby-led feeding has been one of the best and most enjoyable things we have done as a family. It is so much fun watching this little human explore their food and taste new things for the first time. It flies by so take a deep breath and enjoy it. Honestly, the mess gets less and less and before you know it you will have a pro on your hands.

How much should I be feeding my baby?

Don't overload your baby's plate with too much food. Offer small amounts (one mini-muffin at a time, for example) and then look for their cues to see if they are still hungry.

If they are, give them a little more or mix it up by giving them some softly roasted vegetables on the side or some fruit and natural yogurt.

Remember that babies' tummies are much smaller than older children's or grown-ups' and they don't need as much food. They also can fill up easily on bread so make sure you are giving them a varied, colourful diet so they grow up healthy and strong for life!

One of the best things about this way of feeding is that your baby will self-regulate. Once they are full they will just stop eating.

What should my baby be drinking?

If your baby is breastfed then continue to nurse on demand, as your baby gets all the liquid they need from breastmilk.

If you want your little one to start using a sippy cup, you can express a little milk and offer it to them if they are thirsty at mealtimes. As long as your baby is producing regular wet nappies you know they are getting enough liquids.

For babies who are formula fed, you can give them a few sips of cooled boiled water in small amounts, particularly if they are constipated.

Important

Cow's milk is not suitable as a main drink for babies under the age of 12 months. It is OK to use cow's milk for cooking.

Babies and toddlers do not need sugary drinks.

Babies and toddlers do not need juice, as it is full of empty calories.

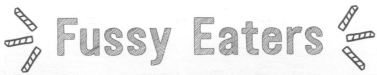

Fussy Eaters

Getting your children to be foodies takes a lot of patience –
a lot! I say this from my own experience. The most important
things I've learned are:

 Babies eat when they are hungry

Your baby may not want to eat their entire
dinner simply because they are not hungry,
and no pleading will get them to eat more.
Just put the food into the fridge and offer it
again in a little while. Usually when they are
hungry enough it will be demolished.

 Be calm and pretend it doesn't bother you

Even if in the back of your mind you are in
anguish about them not eating their broccoli,
just act as if you don't care. Babies are clever
little things and play up to reactions you
have – all three of my kids did. If they saw me
stressed out about carrots, they would refuse
to eat them based on that alone!

 Get the older kids to 'button it'

I have a fussy kid and I know what it's like
to hear him say at dinner, 'I hate asparagus.'
And Oscar wants to be just like his big bro
and copies everything he does. So we had
to have words with the older kids before the
baby decided that he hated it too – we asked
them not to talk about things they didn't like
during meal times, and to just pretend. Now
at dinners Dylan can be heard saying, 'Mmm,
I love this amazing asparagus,' as he winks at
me and his dad. Chancer!

 Eat as a family

I've already mentioned some of the benefits
of this, but besides all the lovely memories
you make, and the fun chats and laughter,
eating together sets a great example for your
baby's eating habits. They see what you are
eating and want to eat the same thing – or,
even funnier, see what their older siblings are
eating and want to impress them by eating
the same thing.

 No alternatives

Refusing to offer alternatives is definitely the
hardest thing to do but it really worked for
me. Dinner times are often my toddler saying
'yuk' to the look of pieces of deliciously
roasted chicken and vegetables or just
pushing his plate into the middle of the
table and breaking into song. He sometimes
refuses to eat and then half an hour later is
pulling at my skirt, looking for a muffin or
cheese on oat crackers. But no, I am a very,
very mean momma and I never cave in. It
takes strength and lots of will power, but
if he doesn't eat his dinner it goes into the
fridge and is offered again when he asks for
something else. Usually it only takes a few
goes of saying, 'Oh, I have your dinner right
here – would you like it now?' for him to say
yes.

Common-Sense
Principles

• ‹‹‹‹∟∟‹‹‹ •

Mother guilt is like a cold – we all get it from time to time. Should we breastfeed or bottle feed? Should we give our babies purées or allow them to feed themselves? Are they eating enough? Are they eating too much? Will my baby be safe eating by himself? Should she be eating more fruit? Is she eating too much fruit?

We have constant concerns about what is best for our little ones and that is part of what makes us great parents. The fact that you're even reading this book means that you want to cook healthy, delicious food for your baby instead of reaching for jars of processed foods.

All of the recipes in this book are the ones I used for my own babies right from the start of their weaning journeys (except for the ones specifically marked for toddlers only). For my own peace of mind, I always make food that can be squashed between my index finger and thumb so I know my little one's gums are strong enough to chew it.

Choking is a really scary word and one that is at the forefront of our thoughts when we start letting our little babies feed themselves. However, once you only offer soft and safe foods, your baby is quite capable of chewing and breaking up the food with their strong gums.

Gagging is a common occurrence in early baby-led feeding, although it might never happen at all. The gag reflex is a safety mechanism that prevents choking as babies learn to move food from the back of their throats to the front. Gagging also teaches them not to stuff their mouths with food. As babies get older and more skilled at eating, they gag less and chew more.

My common-sense principles:

- Make sure your baby is ready! Your baby should be at least six months old, able to sit up unsupported and have good neck strength.

- Tongue thrust should be gone – your baby should have lost the reflex to push foods to the front of their mouth.

- Give foods that are easy to hold – since your baby will be feeding himself/herself, it is important that they are able to pick up foods, hold onto them and get them from their tray to their mouth.

- Don't put food into your baby's mouth (or let anyone else either). Baby-led feeding is letting your baby be in control of what they eat.

- Avoid foods that pose a choking threat, including nuts, whole grapes, whole berries, popcorn and hard chunks of fruit or vegetables.

- Never, ever, ever leave your baby alone when eating.

- Cut small fruits like grapes, blueberries or olives into safe pieces. Grapes should be cut long-ways and I always cut mine into quarters just to be really safe.

- Make sure the food is soft enough. Does it break up if you squeeze it between your index finger and thumb? If so, then your baby should be able to chew it.

- Give your little one time to eat their food – they are small and just learning.

- When your baby is full they will stop eating. Don't try and force them to eat 'one more spoon'.

- If your baby does gag, do not stick your fingers into their mouth or startle them, as this could lead to choking.

According to Gill Rapley, author of *Baby-Led Weaning*, 'provided basic safety rules are observed, choking is no more likely with baby-led weaning than with the conventional method of introducing solids'.

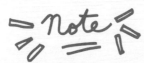 **Note** If you are still worried about what to do if your baby gags or chokes, you could do a course in infant first aid to put your mind at ease.

Being Prepared

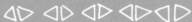

Like most mothers out there, I'm a busy one. We work hard, we pick our babies up from crèche and they want food now! Try telling a hungry eighteen-month-old to wait while you cook him his tea – nope, it just doesn't happen. They don't understand, nor do they care.

Having a freezer drawer filled with yummy goodness has literally saved my sanity. Being able to walk in the door and reheat a muffin or little veggie burger in less than a few minutes really makes such a difference. And if you have forgotten to take a muffin out of the freezer earlier, you can still microwave on a defrost setting. So in less than five minutes of arriving home, your little one can be munching on a healthy meal.

1 Parchment paper is your cleaning saviour!

Using parchment paper under your foods when baking on a tray is the best thing ever. It can just be crumpled up afterwards, thrown into the recycling and you're left with a lovely clean baking tray.

2 Making in bulk

This is one of the best things you can do and it really doesn't take much longer to make 48 muffins, for example, than it does to make 24! Freeze in little bags in your freezer and just grab and go for those busy days. Muffins defrost quickly at room temperature, especially when they are mini ones. The same goes for dinners – make a double dinner and freeze. Just take it out of the freezer the night before and defrost in the fridge overnight, ready to be reheated the next day.

3 Freezing

I try to make the most out of my freezer space. One shelf is for homemade breads, wraps and anything doughy. One shelf is for the baby's little bites. I fill freezer bags with muffins, mini-pies and all things baby-led feeding and those are my go-to foods for lunches, picnics or when I'm out and about. The other shelves are filled with my stash of double dinners, the bags of fruit and veg that I buy in bulk and freeze and, finally, supermarket staples like frozen peas and corn.

- Ideally, frozen food should be covered and defrosted overnight in a suitable container, such as a plate or dish, in the fridge.*

- Only defrost food in a microwave if you are planning to cook the food immediately after it has thawed.*

*Food Safety Authority of Ireland.

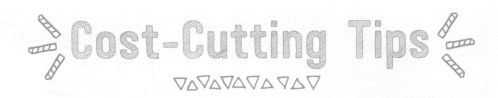

Cost-Cutting Tips

Cost is a huge factor for most families and it is one of the things that holds many of us back when it comes to changing how and what we eat.

I had the perception that eating healthily, especially buying organic food, was going to cost me a fortune but times have really changed. In Ireland, we are so fortunate to have amazing fresh produce right on our doorstep and now even the discount retailers stock organic meats and vegetables at just a few cents more.

The key to eating healthy and spending less money, for me, was cutting out pre-packaged foods. Highly processed foods tend to be the cheaper option but they are also high in salt, sugar and additives, to make them taste like the real deal. The problem is that healthier packaged foods are expensive, so what are we to do? The answer is simple – make your own healthy food. While you may think you draw the line at making something like ketchup, grabbing that bottle in the supermarket for convenience, I promise that in less than five minutes you could have the mixture simmering in the pot and be out in the garden playing ball with your kids. Easy, healthy and inexpensive.

This way of cooking for your baby and your family needs to be accessible to everyone so if you have forked out for an ingredient in this book you will use it again and again in other recipes.

One of the best things about baby-led feeding is that all of the recipes are baby-friendly family meals, so you are not just making food for your little ones and then making an entirely different meal for the rest of the family. You just need to add seasoning to your own plates when serving.

It may seem like work to make everything from scratch but it is really cost effective and healthy for your baby and the entire family. And there is just something about whizzing up your own dips, sauces and treats that makes them taste that little bit nicer.

It also costs far less to feed your little ones like this than it does to buy pre-packaged baby foods. Because your baby is eating tiny portions of what everyone else is eating rather than a different, individual meal, purchased separately, it's far more economical.

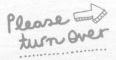

Please turn over

Tips for saving you a few bob!

▽△▽△▽△▽△ ▽△▽

- ### Buy in season
  Look at what vegetables and fruits are in season – it helps to save you money and it supports local farmers. Also, if you have space in your freezer, buy produce in bulk, wash well, then freeze into portioned bags. This is great when organic kale and spinach are in season because you can throw them into things like smoothies, muffins or even stir-fries without having to defrost.

- ### Grow your own
  Let me start by saying that I do not, I repeat, I do not have any green in my fingers. However, putting a few potted herbs (which my husband has to take care of) in our garden has saved me a fortune in buying them. Thyme and rosemary are pretty forgiving in terms of growing, as are chives.

- ### Asian stores
  You will be able to find certain ingredients cheaper in your local Asian store – they're also often sold in large quantities, which can be great value for money. Just search online for Halal store or Asian store to see if you have one in your area.

Ingredients I've found to be great value are:

- **Nuts:** A 1kg bag of almonds will make a lot of almond butter (one of the most expensive nut butters to buy).

- **Medjool dates:** A 1kg box of dates can contain up to 52 dates. That equates to 32.5 portions of my chocolate mousse!

- **Tahini:** A huge tub of tahini will last for ages – unless you're like me and make hummus every few days. In that case, it will probably only last you a month, but you're going to have delicious hummus three times a week at least, so that's pretty OK!

- **Coconut oil:** A large tub of coconut oil lasts for a long time so I only have to buy it every few months.

- **Spices:** It can seem expensive to start a spice collection but they are pretty cheap in Asian stores. The ones you will need most are: cinnamon, nutmeg, cardamom, cumin, coriander, turmeric, paprika and garam masala, so stock up and let's get cooking!

Allergies and Substitutions

When your baby starts weaning, allergies are always a worry – especially when introducing highly allergenic foods like nut butters or eggs. If you or anyone in your family has any reaction to dairy, nuts, shellfish or any other allergen then speak to your health-care provider prior to introducing these foods to your baby.

Gluten

It is important to introduce your baby to gluten before they are seven months old to minimise the risk of coeliac disease. Gluten is found in bread, pasta and cereals and there is no reason not to give these foods to your little one unless they have been diagnosed with a gluten intolerance. If there is already a coeliac in the family, there are some special steps to take before giving your baby gluten. Coeliac Ireland recommend 'offering small amounts of gluten daily from 6 months so that if the disease does develop a blood test would be conclusive'.

Thankfully none of my children have allergies, and we all eat breads and pastas. However, I like to use buckwheat for pancakes, cakes and cookies because it is nutritious and yummy but you can always use regular white flour if you wish.

If your child has been diagnosed with an allergy or if you or your family are vegan and don't want to use dairy, there are many alternatives you can use when making my recipes.

Ingredient	Replace with
1 egg	3 tablespoons flaxseed soaked in 3 tablespoons hot water for a few moments
1 egg	3 tablespoons ground chia seeds in 3 tablespoons of hot water
Cow's milk	Oat milk (use only as a substitute for cooking and not as a main drink)
Butter (dairy)	Avocado, nut butters, coconut oil, olive oil
Wheat flour	Buckwheat flour, coconut flour, oat flour
Nuts	Seeds, beans
Yogurt	Vegan yogurt
Sour cream	Cashew sour cream – soak 200g cashews overnight, drain water, blend until smooth and creamy with the juice of ½ lemon and 1 teaspoon apple cider vinegar.
Gelatine	Agar (available in all good health-food stores)

Sugar, Sugar Everywhere

Sugar is a part of life and you will be hard pressed to find a child who wouldn't bite your hand off for a little bag of chocolates or sugary ice-pop. I myself grew up in a house where a spoonful of sugar actually did make the medicine go down, but things are very different these days.

When we think of sugar, we think of treats – chocolate, sweets and fizzy drinks – but the problem is that most sugars consumed today are hidden in processed foods that aren't classified as desserts or treats. These include breads, sauces, ready-to-eat soups, ready-cooked meals, breakfast cereals and even crackers. Sugar is added to make foods taste more palatable.

Every week there is a new article about research into the disastrous effects that sugar has on our bodies and, more importantly, on our little children. According to the World Health Organization (WHO), Ireland is on course to become the most obese country in Europe and in the coming years we will face an obesity crisis of enormous proportions if we don't act now. The worst part is that our children are the ones being most affected, with the WHO reporting that one in four children are either obese or overweight.

It doesn't help when every second advert on TV entices our children to drink fizzy drinks that will make them smile, eat sweets that will burst flavour into every part of their body and give them energy to be superheroes.

It is also very interesting to know that 1 teaspoon of tomato ketchup contains 1 teaspoon of sugar! And who can really eat just 1 teaspoon of ketchup with a burger and chips? Certainly not most kids I know.

Now is the time to make a change, to support our children's health and to work together to make a difference.

Tips for reducing your family's sugar intake

 ### Encourage eating fresh fruit and vegetables

We all have a sweet tooth, even little babies, who get it from breastmilk. It's a natural thing, but there are ways of satisfying a sweet urge without reaching for highly sugary treats. The healthier snack is *always* fresh fruit or vegetables. The less added sugars we give our children the better.

 ### Make treats occasional

One of the hardest things I find to instil into my children's minds is that treats are for the weekends.

 ### Cook from scratch

Scrap the store-bought jars and opt for making homemade sauces. They are really quick and can also be made in large batches and frozen in ice-cube trays or tubs, ready to be used when you need them.

 ### Lead by example

Babies and toddlers love to copy what their older siblings and parents do, so encourage healthy eating in everyone in your house. It may be a struggle at first but I found baby steps worked for me.

There is nothing wrong with enjoying the occasional treat, but cutting down on sugar will really help make a huge difference in our children's lives.

Maple Syrup

Maple syrup is primarily made of sucrose, which is considered a 'free sugar'. For both adults and children, it is recommended that less than 10% of total daily energy intake comes from free sugar. The free sugar amounts found in *The Baby-Led Feeding Cookbook* recipes don't come close to 5% of total daily energy intake.

According to the World Health Organization and the NHS, the maximum recommended amount of free sugar for children aged four to six years is 19g a day. There are no free sugar recommendations for children under four years of age; however, there is no evidence that less than 5% of total daily energy intake is harmful.

Roisin Gowan
Registered Senior Paediatric Dietitian

Free Sugar in Recipes

Throughout this book, look for the spoon icon, which will show you how much free sugar is in each recipe.

My Kitchen Essentials

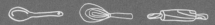

This is not where I tell you to go out and buy a ton of equipment that will, in a few months, end up living in the back of your cupboard, only to be used occasionally. Instead I want to share my 'can't live without' pieces of equipment that help to make these recipes as good as they are.

For the most part your standard kitchen utensils – knives, chopping boards and pans – will suffice, but for nut butters and seed bars you will need a food processor and for sauces, smoothies and soups you will need a blender. Don't confuse the two and try make nut butters, for example, in a blender, as it is not powerful enough and will burn out your motor in no time. Remember that you need liquid for a blender but not for a food processor.

Food processor

My mother received a Kenwood mixer as a wedding present forty years ago and to this day she still uses it, so it was engrained in me to invest in my own. I bought a Kenwood Multipro and it was worth every cent. It slices, grates, makes nut butters and also comes with a blender which, as a whole, will save you money on buying both.

NutriBullet

We have used our NutriBullet every single day for the past year. It is a powerful little machine that blends even the tiniest of seeds into a delicious smoothie in less than a minute. Not only that, it is so easy to use that my nine-year-old can rock in from school, throw some spinach, a banana and a few strawberries into it and he has a healthy smoothie. The NutriBullet is also great for making flours – mine came with a milling blade – so just add 100g of rolled oats, whizz up for one minute and you have oat flour. It also works for nuts and seeds, which is perfect for little weaning babies.

Spiraliser

This is great for making noodles out of vegetables. If you don't want to buy one you can buy a julienne peeler instead, which does the same thing – it just takes more time.

Mini-muffin tin

My favourite baby-led feeding utensil is my mini-muffin tin. I love it and use it most days, either to cook or portion and freeze bite-sized meals for my little one. They are pretty easy to find in most stores but just make sure you get a good non-stick one!

Pestle and mortar

Buying a pestle and mortar is relatively inexpensive and it will come in really useful for grinding down nuts, spices and wholegrains which otherwise would be dangerous for little babies.

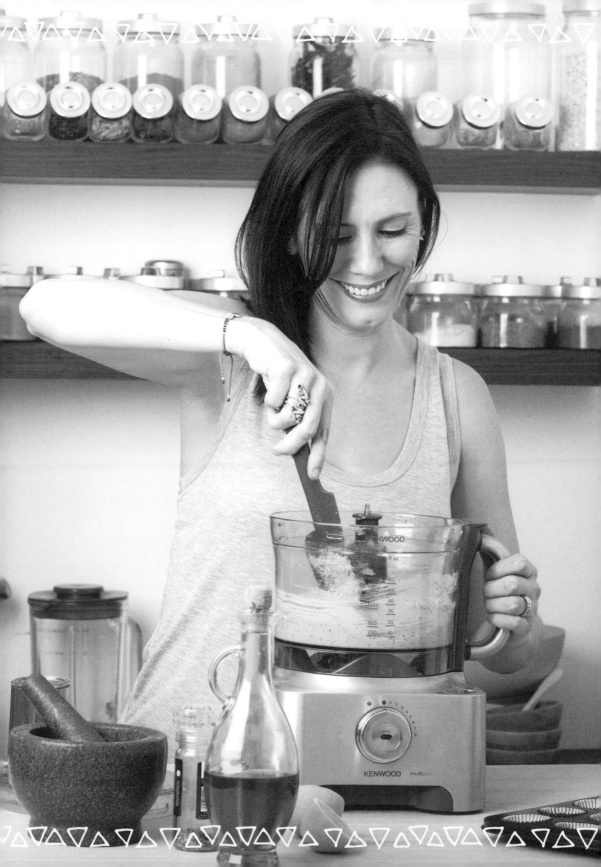

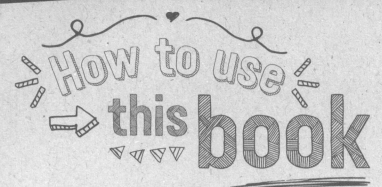

How to use this book

1.
Offer **small amounts** and watch your baby's cues to see if they want more. They will stop eating when they are full!

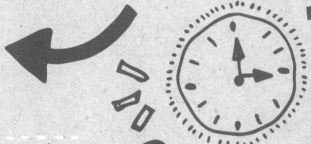

2.
Add a side of soft **veggies** or **fruit** to recipes for even more **yummy goodness.**

3.
Eat as a family at normal meal times. Breakfast, lunch and *dinner*

5.
A little sip of water is OK so babies learn to drink from a cup. A baby's main drink should only be breastmilk or formula until they are 12 months old.

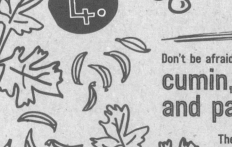

4.
Don't be afraid of spices like **cumin, coriander and paprika.**

They add lots of yummy flavours for babies.

SIPPY CUP

6.

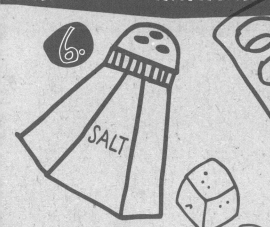

SALT

Salt & refined Sugar

refined

are not needed for babies.

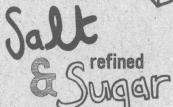

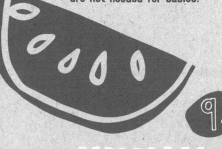

9.

Be treat-wise by making the natural and yummy treats and snacks for your entire family. If your older kiddies are munching away on healthy chocolate-covered watermelon then the baby will want it too!

7.

... Batch Cook

Cook double breakfasts, dinners and lunches and then freeze them so you always have yummy food on hand for your baby.

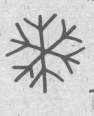

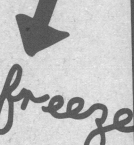

freeze

8.

Most dishes in this book can be frozen, making it convenient for busy mums and dads.

10. Keep trying if your baby says

Yuk!

It can take at least

10 tries

for your baby to learn to

love

food they dislike initially.

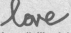

All eggs are large and free range.
All butter is unsalted.
All vanilla extract is sugar free.
All seeds are milled.
All milk is full fat.

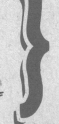

NOTE

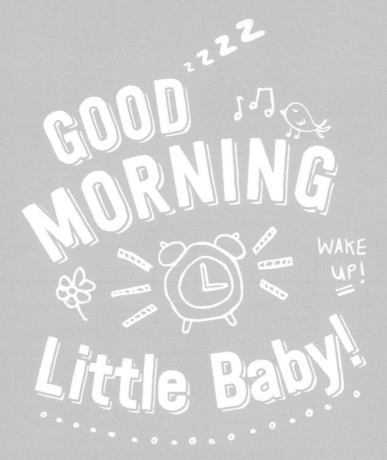

After (hopefully) a good night's sleep, your little one will wake up hungry for a **delicious breakfast.**

Start their day off the right way by filling their tummies with **nutritious goodness,** giving them bundles of energy to do all the things a little baby should. I have included recipes for busy mornings when you need something quick and handy, as well as for relaxed weekends when you have a little more time on your hands.

Three-Ingredient
Banana Pancakes

Three-ingredient pancakes for those mornings you want to whip up something quick yet satisfying for your little one. Given the small amount of ingredients, you might think these little pancakes would be boring, but they are deliciously fluffy and naturally sweet. They freeze well and reheat in the toaster so are an ideal breakfast for busy mornings.

Makes 12 pancakes

2 bananas, peeled
3 eggs
1 teaspoon baking powder
rapeseed oil for frying

In a blender, blend the bananas until they are smooth and completely creamy.

In a separate bowl, whisk the eggs with the baking powder and then fold in the puréed banana.

Heat a frying pan and add about a teaspoon of oil per batch. Spoon 2–3 tablespoons of batter per pancake into the pan. Cook until you see bubbles forming (about 1–2 minutes). Flip over and cook the other side.

Serve with fresh fruit and, for an extra treat, drizzle with a little maple syrup.

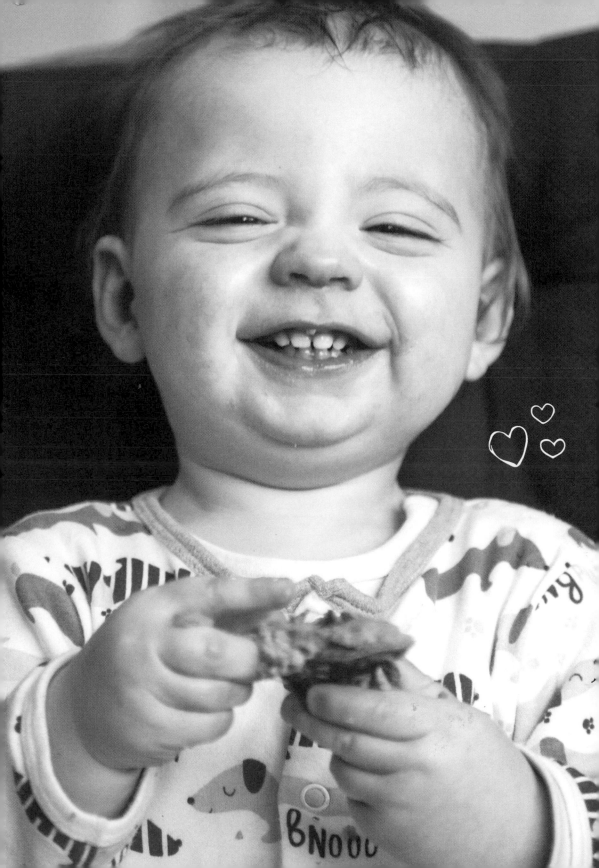

Ginger Buckwheat Pancakes with Caramelised Coconut Pears

Light and fluffy pancakes with delicious caramelised pear and ginger will start your family's morning off with a smile. These pancakes are a take on one of the most popular recipes from my blog, and they are so good you will end up making them every weekend.

Makes 12 pancakes

120g buckwheat flour

2 teaspoons baking powder

250ml milk

1 egg

2 tablespoons melted unsalted butter

2 teaspoons vanilla extract

rapeseed oil for frying

For the topping

1 tablespoon coconut oil

1 pear, finely sliced

2 tablespoons ginger root, grated

maple syrup, to serve

Add buckwheat flour and baking powder to a mixing bowl.

In a separate jug, mix the milk, egg, melted butter and vanilla.

Make a well in the middle of the flour and slowly whisk the liquid mixture in until smooth and completely combined.

For each batch of pancakes, heat ½ a teaspoon of rapeseed oil in a large frying pan over a medium heat. Spoon 2–3 tablespoons of batter per pancake into the pan. Cook until you see bubbles forming (about 1–2 minutes). Flip over and cook the other side.

To make the topping, heat the coconut oil in a pan. Add the pear and cook on both sides until it starts to brown slightly. Add the ginger and cook for a few moments.

To serve the pancakes, spoon the pear and ginger over. Drizzle with a little maple syrup.

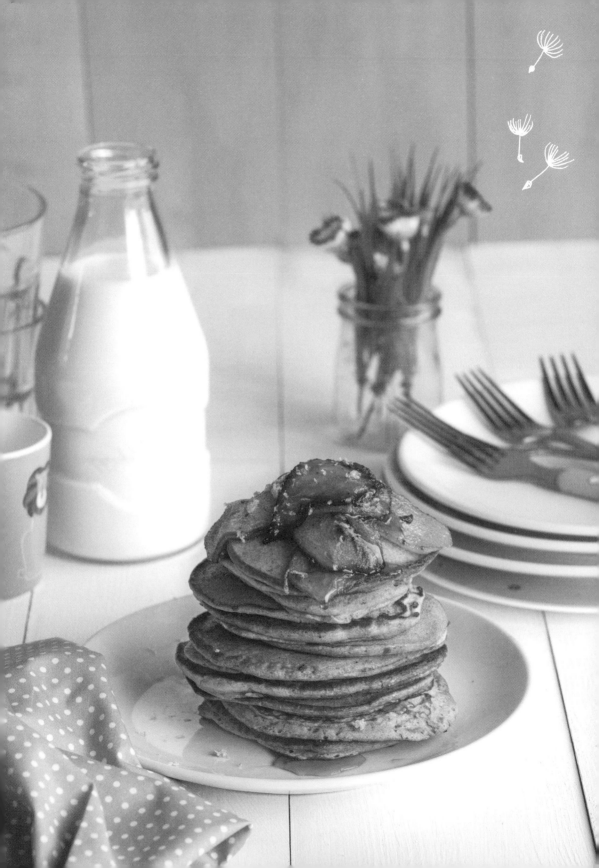

Blueberry Baked Pancakes

Baked pancakes can be a huge time saver. There is no flipping and tossing while a baby pulls at your legs, wondering when breakfast will be served. The texture is more like a fairy cake than a pancake. They are deliciously light and perfect for baby hands.

Makes 24 pancakes

2 tbsp (40g): 24.2g free sugar
(24 servings) 1.0g each

150g plain flour
2 teaspoons baking powder
250ml milk
1 egg
2 tablespoons unsalted butter, melted
2 tablespoons maple syrup
48 blueberries

Preheat oven to 180°C/350°F/gas 4.

Add flour and baking powder to a mixing bowl.

In a separate jug, mix together the milk, egg, melted unsalted butter and maple syrup.

Make a well in the middle of your flour mixture and slowly whisk the liquid mixture into the flour until smooth and completely combined.

Pour into an oiled mini-muffin tin, add 2 blueberries to each and bake for 25 minutes or until the pancakes have risen and are golden.

Blueberry & Custard
Bread Pudding

As a child, one of my favourite desserts was bread pudding. It always reminds me of my grandad, sitting by his side as we spooned piping hot pudding to our lips, blowing to cool it down before demolishing a whole bowl of it. I hope he would approve of my sugar-free, egg-free, banana-and-blueberry-sweetened version. Oscar does – so I'm pretty sure Grandad would agree!

Makes 24

250ml milk

1 banana

1 tablespoon cornflour

1 teaspoon vanilla

125g blueberries

200g bread, finely chopped

Preheat oven to 180°C/350°F/gas 4.

To make the custard, blend the milk and banana until completely smooth and then pour into a saucepan. Warm over a medium heat until piping hot but not boiling and then reduce to a simmer.

In a cup or small bowl, mix the cornflour with 1 tablespoon of water until it becomes a paste and then slowly pour it into the banana and milk, whisking as you do. Cook for about 3 minutes on a medium heat, stirring regularly, until the milk starts to thicken. Remove from the heat.

Add the vanilla, blueberries and bread to the pan and stir for a minute or two until the bread is completely soggy and has soaked up a lot of the custard.

Spoon the mixture into an oiled mini-muffin tin and bake for 25 minutes or until the tops are golden. Allow to cool before removing from the tin. Serve warm or cold.

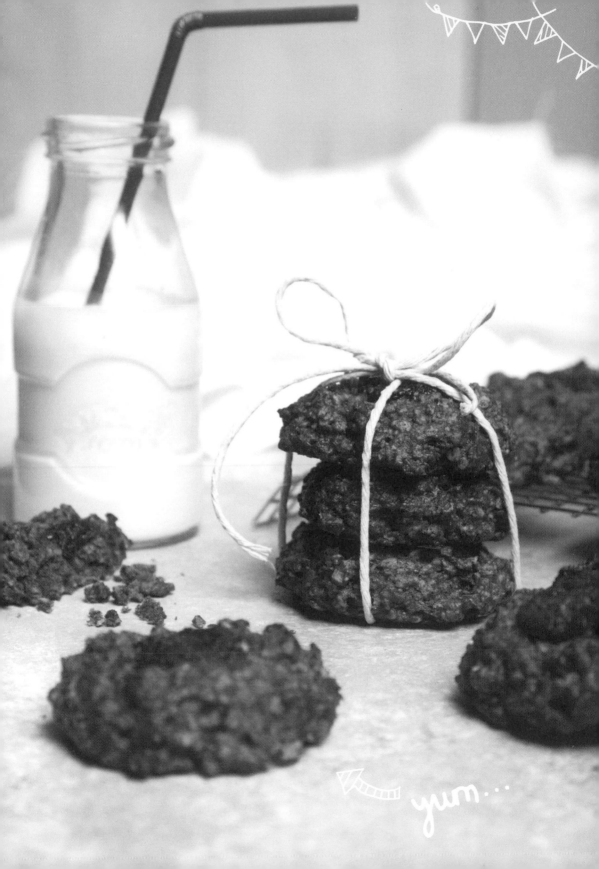

yum...

Good Morning Baby
Breakfast Cookies

Cookies for breakfast? Who ever heard of such a thing! You can whip up a batch of these in less than 5 minutes and the smell alone, wafting down the hallway, will be enough to wake anyone up. They are my take on a healthy breakfast bar, using wholefoods, no sugar and only fruit to make them sweet. They taste so amazing that they barely ever make it past one day before they are eaten in our house.

Makes 16 cookies

3 ripe bananas

60ml rapeseed or olive oil

160g peanut butter

200g oats

1 teaspoon bicarbonate of soda

1 teaspoon ground ginger

1 teaspoon ground cinnamon

1 teaspoon vanilla extract

4 tablespoons Chia Jam (see page 193)

Preheat oven to 160°C/325°F/gas 3.

Add the bananas, oil and peanut butter to your blender and blend until smooth and gooey.

Place all of the remaining ingredients (except for the chia jam) into a bowl and pour the banana mixture in. Stir until completely combined.

Spoon a heaped tablespoon of the mixture per cookie onto a lightly oiled baking tray. Leave a little space between each one.

Using the back of the spoon, press down the centre of each cookie to make a little well; then place about a teaspoon of Chia Jam into each one.

Bake in the oven for 12–15 minutes. Keep an eye on them from 12 minutes on, as you don't want them to get too hard for little mouths.

Remove from the oven and leave to cool and set before giving them to your baby.

Spinach &
Eggy Bread Bites

What better way to start your baby's day than with spinach, egg and bread all muddled up together and baked into little bites of yumminess. This recipe is better if prepared the night before, as it gives the wet mixture a chance to soak properly into the bread. Perfect for little hands to hold and will be devoured by the entire family – just you wait.

Makes 24 bites

1 tablespoon rapeseed or olive oil

1 small onion, diced

2 cloves garlic, crushed

100g spinach, chopped

200g bread, diced

6 eggs

80ml milk

sprig of rosemary, leaves picked and chopped

¼ teaspoon black pepper

Preheat oven to 160°C/325°F/gas 3.

Heat the oil in a pan and gently fry the onion over a medium heat until soft and sticky. Add the garlic and fry for a further 2–3 minutes until cooked but not browned. Add the chopped spinach, stir for about 30 seconds, then remove the pan from the heat.

Place the diced bread in a bowl and add the spinach, onion and garlic mixture.

Whisk the eggs and milk in a jug until creamy and then pour over the bread and spinach mixture. Sprinkle in the rosemary and pepper and give everything a good stir. The bread should be totally coated.

Cover with cling film and leave in the fridge for a few hours or overnight.

Spoon into a well-oiled mini-muffin tin and bake for 25 minutes until golden brown. Allow to cool slightly before serving.

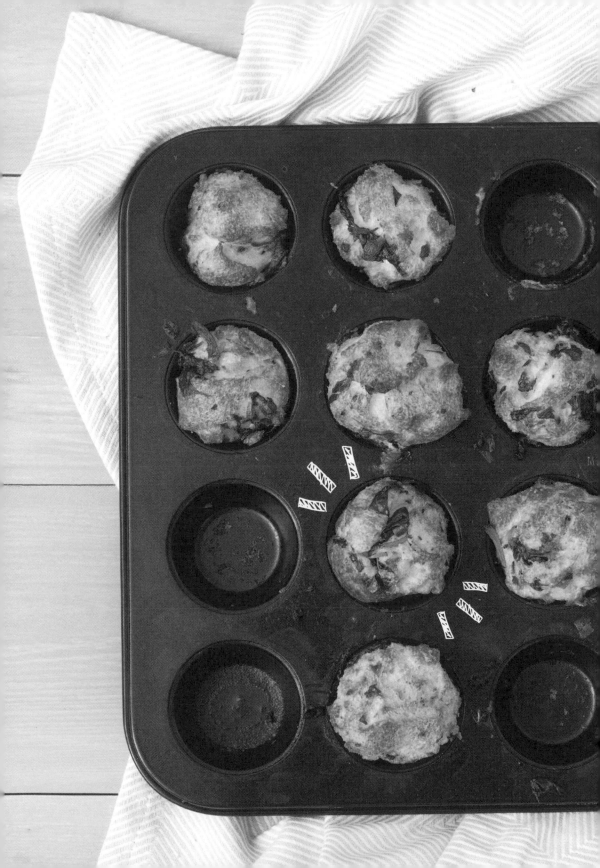

Mango, Coconut & Turmeric
Chia Seed Pudding

Using chia seeds to make an overnight pudding is a great way to introduce them to your baby's diet. Overnight, they expand to soak up all the liquid, making them easily digestible for little tummies. This chia pudding is yummy and babies love it! Use pre-loaded spoons for smaller weaning babies, as it can be quite messy otherwise.

Serves 2 adults and 2 children

400ml coconut milk

1 banana

4 tablespoons chia seeds

1 teaspoon vanilla extract

¼ teaspoon ground cinnamon

1 medium-sized mango, peeled, stoned and roughly chopped

½ teaspoon turmeric

slices of dragon fruit, to serve

Place the coconut milk and banana in a blender and whizz until smooth and silky. Pour into a jug and add the chia seeds, vanilla and cinnamon. Stir well to ensure the mixture is fully combined.

Divide about half of the mixture between 4 small bowls or jars, leaving the remaining chia seed mixture in the jug. Leave in the fridge for at least 4 hours but preferably overnight.

When you are ready to serve, blend the fresh mango with turmeric until smooth. Spoon 2 tablespoons of this mixture into each bowl or jar, then fill them up with the remaining chia pudding mixture from the jug. Finish with another spoon of mango and add a piece of dragon fruit to the top for extra flavour.

Keeps in the fridge for about 3–4 days. Leftovers can be frozen and defrosted in the fridge overnight.

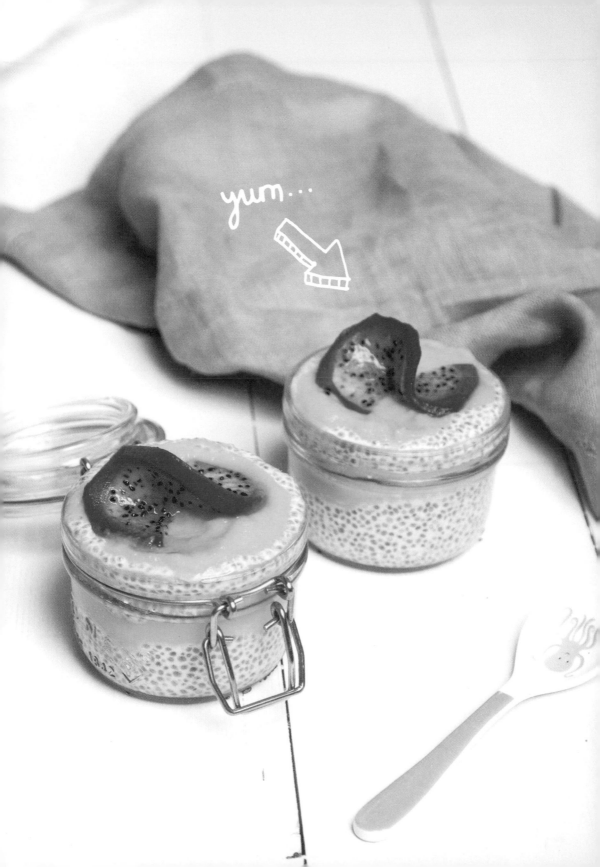

yum…

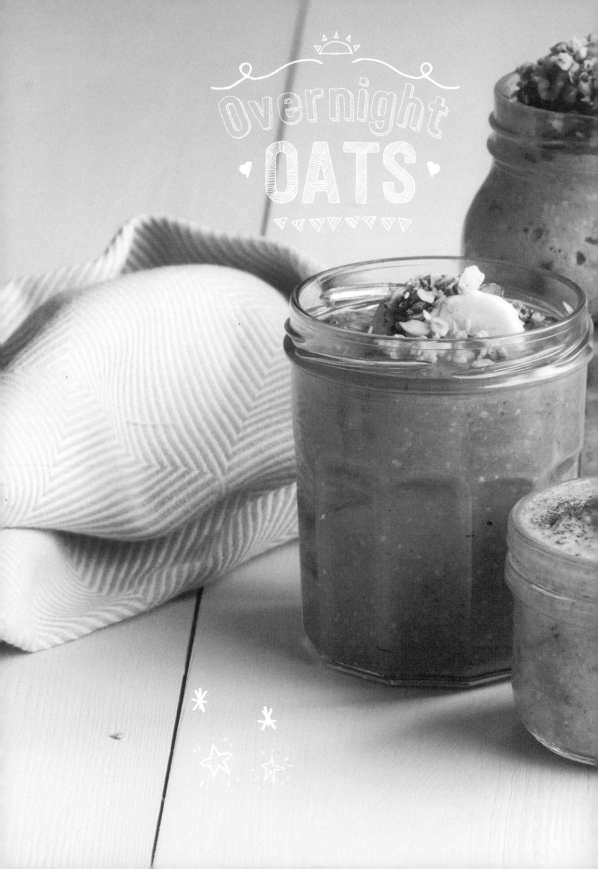

overnight
OATS

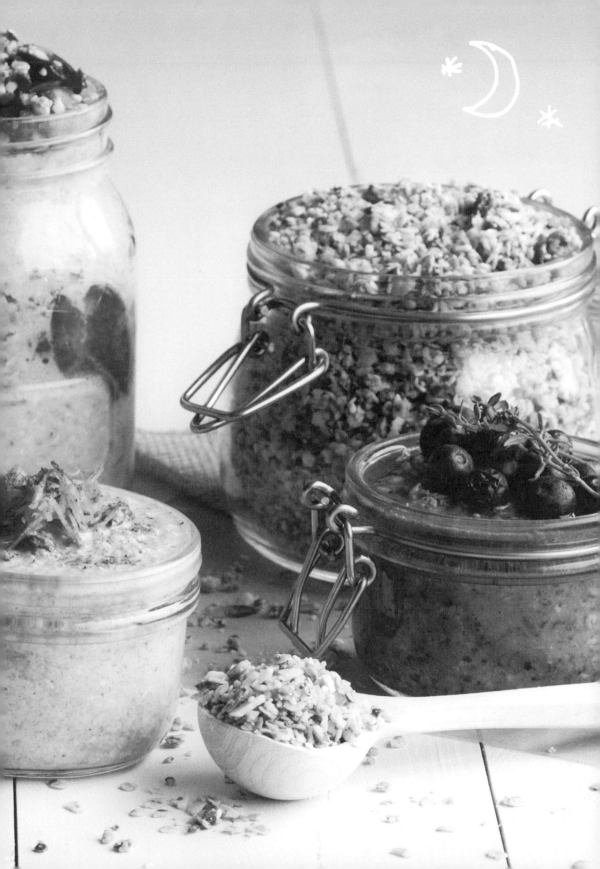

Overnight Oats
4 Ways

When I first discovered overnight oats I thought I was a genius. That was until I went onto Pinterest and realised so had half the world! Children love them because they not only look pretty, but also taste like a dessert – you'll never have to utter 'eat your porridge' again. For smaller little ones who cannot yet manage a spoon, just pour the mixture into a lightly oiled mini-muffin tin and bake for 25 minutes to form bite-sized oat muffins.

Each recipe serves 2 adults and 2 children

2 tsp (10g) : 6g free sugar
(4 servings) 1.5g each

Carrot Cake Overnight Oats

250ml almond milk

50g grated carrot, plus extra for decoration

1 teaspoon vanilla extract

15 raisins

2 teaspoons maple syrup

3 tablespoons natural yogurt

pinch of ground cinnamon

pinch of nutmeg

100g oats

Add all of the ingredients except the oats to a blender and blend until smooth and creamy.

Place oats in a jar or bowl and pour the milk mixture over. Stir well, cover and place in the fridge overnight.

To serve, sprinkle a little grated carrot and a little extra cinnamon on top.

Strawberry Shortcake Overnight Oats

250ml almond milk

6 large strawberries, 3 sliced, for decorating

2 teaspoons vanilla extract

2 teaspoons maple syrup

100g oats

Add almond milk, 3 strawberries, vanilla and maple syrup to a blender and blend until smooth and silky.

Add oats to a jar or bowl and pour the milk and strawberry mixture over them. Give it a good stir, then add the sliced strawberries on top. Cover and leave in the fridge overnight.

Serve with some Baby Fine Granola (see page 42) sprinkled on top.

Chocolate and Banana Overnight Oats

250ml almond milk

2 Medjool dates

1 heaped teaspoon cacao

1 banana

125ml natural yogurt

2 teaspoons vanilla extract

100g oats

Add almond milk, dates, cacao, banana and vanilla to a blender and blend until completely smooth.

Place the oats in a jar or bowl, pour the milk and banana mixture over, add the yogurt and stir well. Cover and leave in the fridge overnight.

Serve with sliced banana and Baby Fine Granola (see page 42).

Blueberry and Thyme Overnight Oats

250ml almond milk

1 teaspoon fresh thyme leaves, finely chopped

1 teaspoon vanilla extract

2 teaspoons maple syrup

150g blueberries, plus extra to serve

100g oats

Add almond milk, thyme, vanilla, maple syrup and blueberries to a blender and blend until smooth and creamy.

Add oats to a bowl or jar and pour the milk mixture on top. Stir well, cover and place in the fridge overnight.

To serve, top with some fresh blueberries and a sprinkle of fresh thyme.

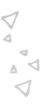

Baby Fine Granola

Granola makes a perfect snack for babies – and even grown-up kids of all ages. When you see how easy it is to make, you will never buy the sugary store-bought kind again. This recipe uses ingredients that are nourishing and delicious. The seeds are pulsed a few times, making them just the right consistency for little ones. Serve over natural yogurt and fresh berries for the ultimate snack!

Makes 24 Servings

60ml: 36.3g free sugar
(24 servings) 1.5g each

40g pumpkin seeds

40g sunflower seeds

30g goji berries

60g toasted almond flakes

200g oats

60ml maple syrup

80g coconut oil, melted

2 tablespoons sesame seeds

Preheat the oven to 140°C/275°F/gas 1.

Add pumpkin seeds, sunflower seeds, goji berries and almond flakes to a food processor and pulse a few times until the seeds are broken up into smaller, manageable baby-sized pieces.

Pour the mixture into a large bowl and add all of the remaining ingredients. Using your hands, mix it all together, making sure the oats are fully coated and sticky.

Line a large baking tray with parchment paper and spread the mixture evenly and loosely, making sure there are no clumps.

Bake for 10 minutes, then remove the tray from the oven, mix the granola around again and bake for a further 10 minutes. The granola should be slightly golden and not too crunchy.

Store in an airtight jar.

Baked Porridge
& Apple Muffins

I couldn't do this book justice without including these muffins. They have been the most popular recipe on my blog to date and so many babies all over the world have tried and loved them. For smaller babies, they are the perfect food to start their weaning journey, as they are easy for little hands to manage and are also very nutritious.

Makes 24 mini-muffins

60ml: 36.3g free sugar
(24 servings) 1.5g each

100g oats

4 tablespoons raisins

1 teaspoon ground cinnamon

½ teaspoon ground nutmeg

2 eggs, beaten

300ml milk

1 apple, chopped into small pieces

2 tablespoons sunflower seeds, finely ground

1 tablespoon chia seeds

First soak your oats overnight – place in a bowl and cover with water. They are so much lighter and fluffier when you do this. The next morning, drain before using.

Preheat the oven to 180°C/350°F/gas 4.

In a large bowl, mix all the ingredients together.

Spoon into an oiled mini-muffin tin and bake for 20–25 mins or until golden brown.

At the weekend, we serve ours with a tiny drizzle of maple syrup.

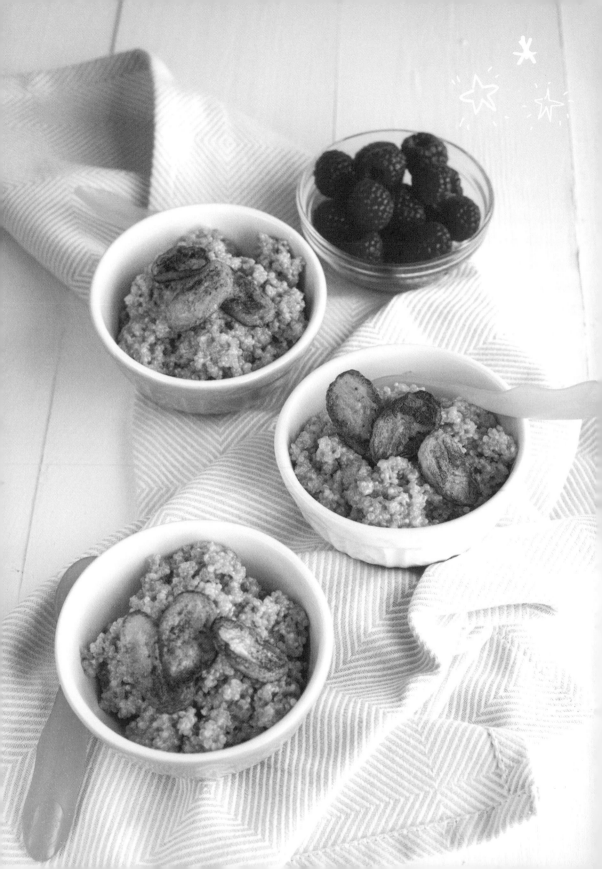

Quinoa Porridge with
Caramelised Banana & Raspberries

Quinoa is a wonder grain. It is an excellent source of protein and fibre, which makes it ideal for breakfast when you want to give your little one something really filling and delicious.

Serves 2 adults and 2 children

2 tbsp (40g): 24.2g free sugar
(4 servings) 6g each

100g quinoa

250ml oat milk

60ml coconut milk

2 teaspoons vanilla extract

2 tablespoons maple syrup

2 tablespoons coconut oil

2 bananas, sliced

12 fresh raspberries

Place the quinoa into a sieve and wash under cold running water until it runs clear.

Pour it into a saucepan with the oat milk. Cook over a medium heat, stirring all the time. The quinoa should thicken and absorb all of the milk.

Remove from the heat and stir in the coconut milk, vanilla and maple syrup until it is creamy, then pour into bowls.

Melt the coconut oil in a frying pan over a medium heat and add the sliced banana. Fry both sides until they are caramelised. Place on top of the quinoa and serve with some fresh raspberries.

Baked French Toast
with Raspberries

This is such a simple morning recipe but it tastes so yummy it feels like a treat. I leave the bread soaking overnight and pop it in the oven on those busy mornings when we want something tasty but don't have much time.

Serves 2 adults and 2 children

1 tbsp (20g): 12.1g free sugar
(4 servings) 3g each

250g good quality bread, cut into small cubes

6 eggs

1 tablespoon maple syrup

125ml milk

¼ teaspoon ground cinnamon

1 tablespoon vanilla extract

250g raspberries

Preheat oven to 180°C/350°F/gas 4.

Place the bread in a bowl.

In a separate bowl, whisk the eggs with the maple syrup, milk, cinnamon and vanilla until light and creamy and then pour over the bread.

Spoon into 4 well-buttered, individual tart tins and top each one with some of the fresh raspberries. If you don't have small tart tins, you can put the entire mixture in a large baking dish.

Bake for 25 minutes until starting to turn golden.

Serve warm.

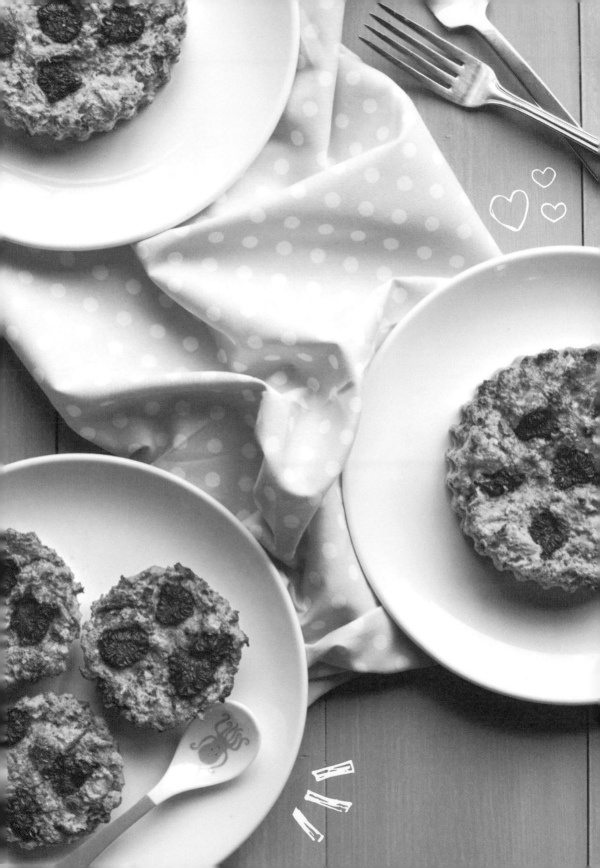

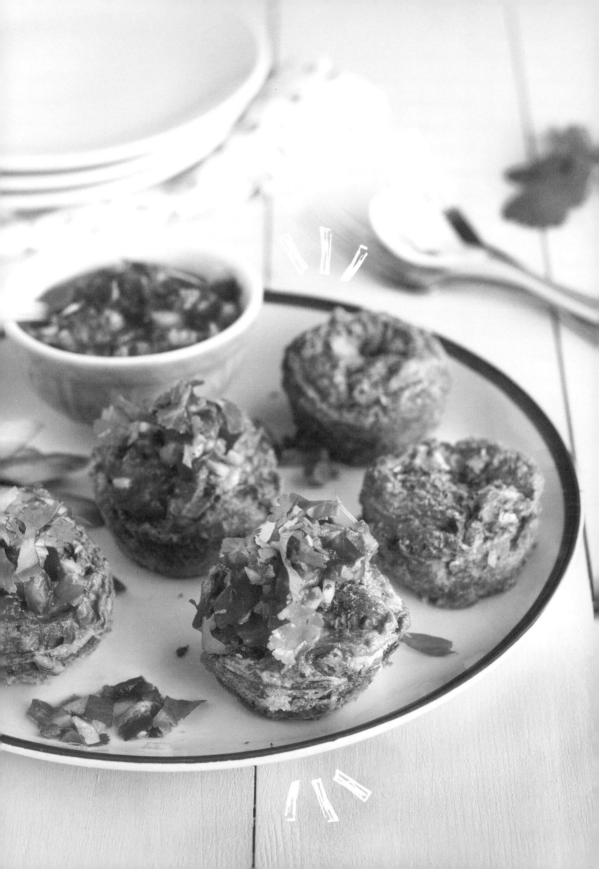

Huevos Rancheros –
Baked Mexican Eggs in Bread

There is nothing like eggs for breakfast, and with some Mexican spices they totally come to life! I prepare the eggs and salsa the night before to save on time. It's so good with some chunky guacamole – or, for little hands, spears of delicious avocado.

Makes 12

6 slices of bread

butter for greasing

6 eggs

½ teaspoon ground cumin

½ teaspoon ground coriander

½ teaspoon paprika

½ teaspoon ground cinnamon

¼ teaspoon chilli powder (optional)

small bunch fresh coriander, finely chopped

Preheat oven to 190°C/375°F/gas 5.

Roll each slice of bread out with a rolling pin until really flat and then cut in half. Butter a regular-sized muffin tin and line each cup with half a slice of bread.

In a mixing bowl, whisk the egg with the remaining ingredients and pour into the bread bowls.

Bake for 25 minutes or until the egg is totally set.

Serve with homemade salsa and guacamole (see page 201).

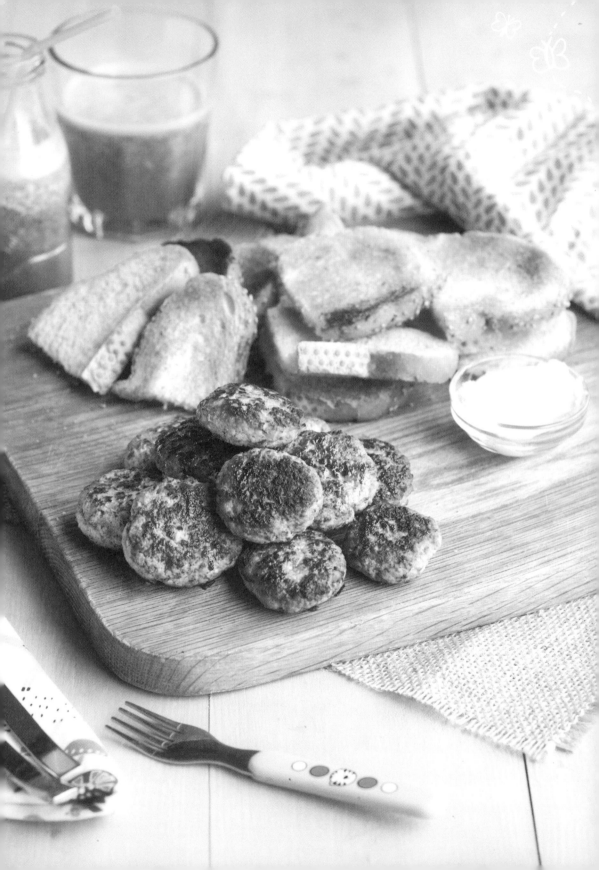

Sausage Patties
with Apple and Pork

Store-bought sausages can be full of additives and also high in salt, so I wanted to make a healthy version. I shaped these into small patties so they are safe for little mouths and the perfect size for little hands.

Makes 24 patties

320g lean pork mince

¼ teaspoon ground cumin

2 teaspoons thyme, finely chopped

2 teaspoons rosemary leaves, finely chopped

¼ teaspoon ground black pepper

1 egg

4 tablespoons breadcrumbs

50g grated apple

rapeseed oil, for frying

Add all of the ingredients except the oil to a bowl and mix really well.

Using your hands, shape tablespoons of the mixture into small patties and flatten down slightly.

Heat some rapeseed oil in a pan over a medium heat and gently fry the patties on each side until golden. You can also grill them until golden and cooked through.

Serve with toast and a green smoothie for a delicious breakfast.

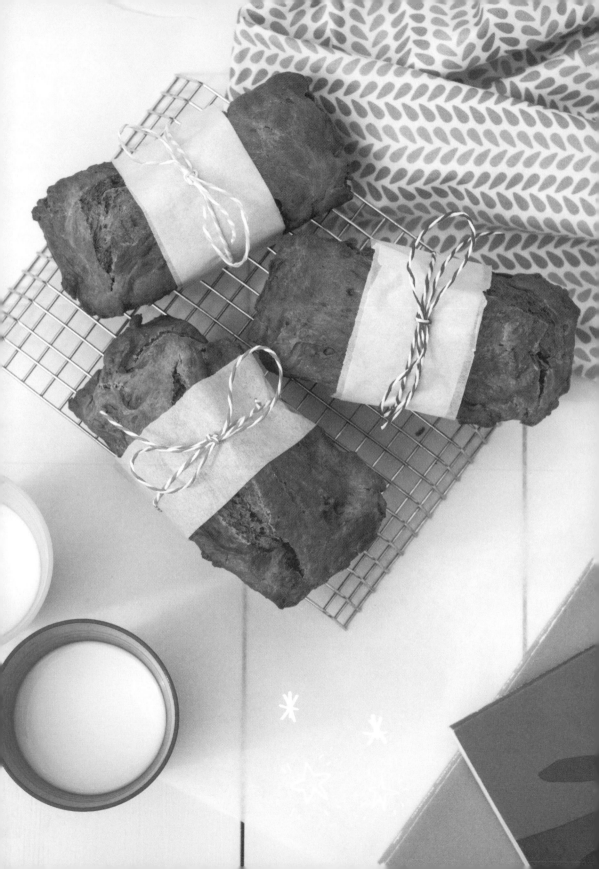

Baby Banana Bread

Bananas are so amazingly sweet that they don't need any added sugar to create a delicious bread. The darker, blacker fruits work best, as they become sweeter with age. This bread is light, fluffy and flavoursome and makes a super alternative to ordinary bread.

Makes 3 mini-loaves (15 x 8.5cm)

4 large, very ripe bananas, mashed

2 eggs, beaten

2 tablespoons melted unsalted butter

1 teaspoon ground cinnamon

1 teaspoon vanilla extract

2 teaspoons bicarbonate of soda

2 tablespoons olive oil

240g plain flour

Preheat oven to 160°C/325°F/gas 3.

Place mashed bananas in a bowl, then add the remaining ingredients and stir until fully combined.

Pour into 3 mini-loaf tins lined with parchment paper.

Bake for about 50 minutes or until a skewer inserted in the loaves comes out clean.

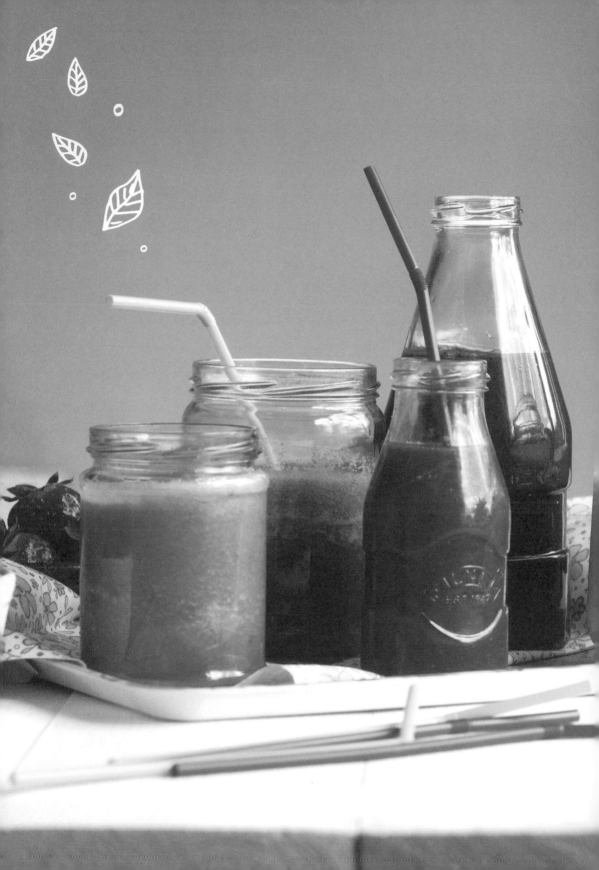

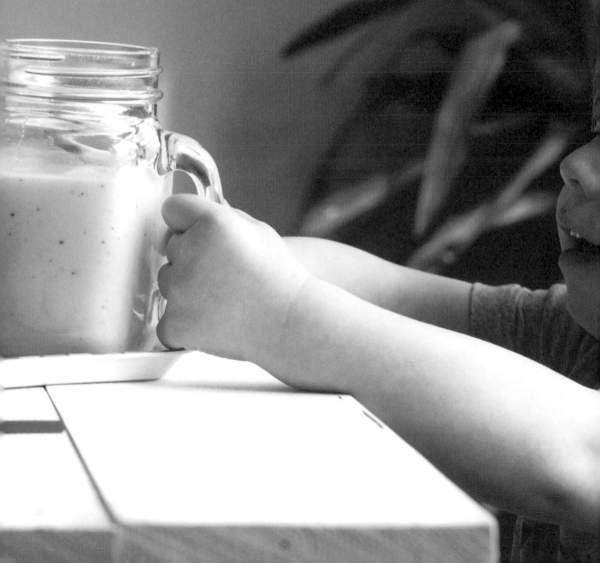
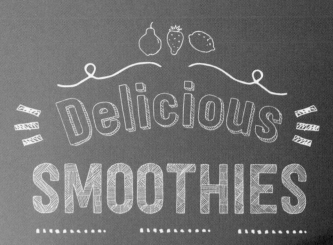

Delicious SMOOTHIES

Smoothies
for You & Baby

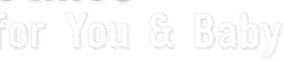

Smoothies are a great way to get some extra vitamins and minerals into little ones when they are having those 'off-food' days from teething or sickness. I try to use mostly vegetables, sweetened with fruit, to make them even healthier.

For each recipe, simply pop all the ingredients into a blender and blend until smooth. Drink straight away or pour into baby-sized ice-pop moulds and freeze – perfect for teething gums!

Each recipe makes 1 adult and 1 baby smoothie

The Yellow One

I have to give credit to my mango-loving husband for this recipe. It is amazing how such simple ingredients can make something so wonderful.

1 ready-to-eat mango, peeled and roughly chopped
2 passion fruit, flesh only
2 tablespoons natural yogurt
250ml milk
½ teaspoon turmeric

The Orange One

This is one of my favourite smoothies: orange and carrot blended together with a little pineapple and coconut water. It's full of vitamin C and beta-carotene (from all those carrots) and will have your little bunny hopping around in no time.

120g carrot, washed, topped and tailed and roughly chopped
120g fresh pineapple, peeled and roughly chopped
½ whole orange
320ml coconut water

The Red One

The combination of vegetables in this smoothie might put you off, but I promise you it tastes so good! Red peppers are deliciously sweet and juicy, as are tomatoes, and when blended up with berries and coconut water you won't even know they are there.

1 ripe tomato, roughly chopped

80g red pepper, roughly chopped

6 ripe strawberries

1 banana

1 tablespoon goji berries

320ml coconut water

The Purple One

Berries are little powerhouses of nutrients and vitamins and are also full of antioxidants, so you can imagine how good this smoothie is for you – and it's blended up with my favourite vegetable, beetroot. It's full of flavour and the little ones love it!

60g blueberries

60g blackberries

30g kale

1 medium raw beetroot, washed and roughly chopped

320ml coconut water

The Green One

A smoothie so powerful it should really come with its own theme song. Yes, it is psychedelic green in colour but that's what superheroes like to drink, don't you know ... This is my go-to smoothie when my little ones are under the weather, as it has so much goodness packed into a delicious drink.

50g kale

1 lime, juice only

70g cucumber, washed and roughly chopped

30g celery, washed and roughly chopped

1 green apple, washed and roughly chopped

5g fresh ginger root, peeled

320ml coconut water

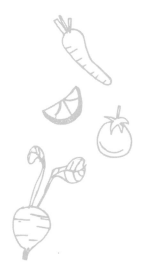

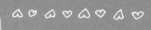

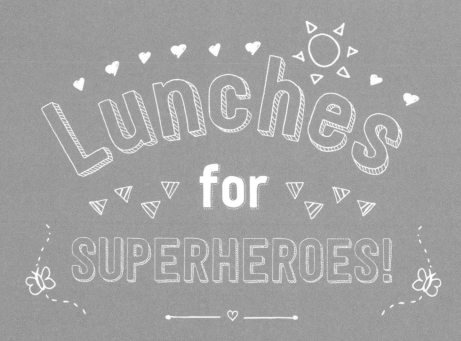

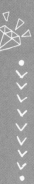
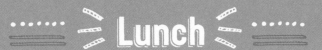

Lunch

is one of your baby's three main meals of the day, so it is important to refuel them with **delicious and healthy** food. Many of these recipes can be made ahead of time and stored in the freezer, making life a bit easier for busy mums and dads. There is something here to suit every kind of day – from sunny picnics in the park to cold, wet winter afternoons indoors.

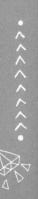

Super-Quick Tomato Soup

Nothing beats a warm, delicious soup that takes less than 15 minutes to prepare, including blending and pouring into bowls. The smooth texture of this soup is like a hug in mug. Deliciously warming and full of goodness.

Serves 2 adults and 2 children

2 tablespoons olive oil

2 red onions, chopped

2 cloves garlic, crushed

4 tablespoons unsalted tomato purée

800g tinned plum tomatoes

1 litre homemade vegetable stock

black pepper, to season

1 tablespoon fresh oregano, chopped

1 tablespoon fresh parsley, chopped

125ml natural yogurt

Heat the olive oil in a large saucepan over a medium heat, then add the onions. Cook for about 8 minutes until sweet and caramelised. Add the garlic and cook for a further 2–3 minutes.

Add the tomato purée, tins of tomatoes and stock to the saucepan and stir well. Season with pepper, then turn the heat down to low.

When the soup starts to bubble, remove from the heat, add the oregano and ¾ of the parsley and then, using a stick blender, blend until smooth and creamy.

Serve with a little natural yogurt and the rest of the fresh parsley scattered on top.

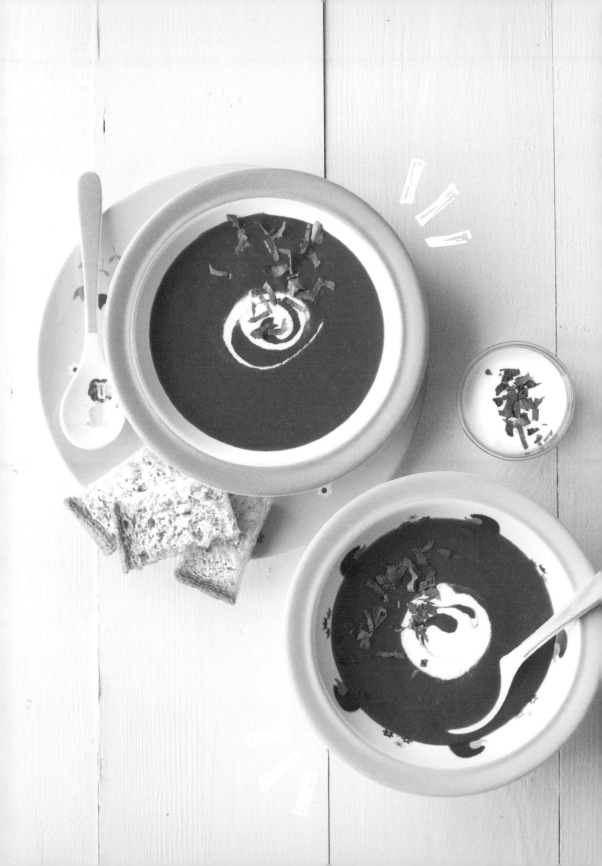

Mexican
Bean Stew

It is actually quite easy for babies to eat this soup. When it's cooked, you can separate the broth from the vegetables, pour the broth into a sippy cup and leave the vegetables and beans in your little one's bowl. Then they can get to work picking up and sipping in their own time. This soup is zingy and has such a delicious taste that we seldom have any leftovers for the freezer.

Serves 2 adults and 2 children

2 tablespoons rapeseed oil

1 large red onion, chopped

4 cloves garlic, thinly sliced

4 tablespoons tomato purée

400g tinned chopped tomatoes

800ml homemade chicken stock (see page 205)

800g tinned black beans

200g corn kernels (frozen or tinned)

1 teaspoon ground coriander

1 teaspoon ground cumin

1 teaspoon ground paprika

1 lime, juice only

small bunch fresh coriander, finely chopped, to serve

natural yogurt, to serve

Heat the rapeseed oil in a large saucepan. Add the chopped onion and fry until it becomes soft. Add the garlic, give it a good stir and allow to cook for a further 2–3 minutes until the garlic is soft but not browned.

Add the tomato purée and stir well, then add the tinned tomatoes, stock, black beans, corn, spices and lime juice and stir well. Turn the heat to low and simmer for 15 minutes.

To serve, ladle the soup into bowls, then sprinkle the fresh coriander on top. Add a dollop of natural yogurt to the middle and enjoy!

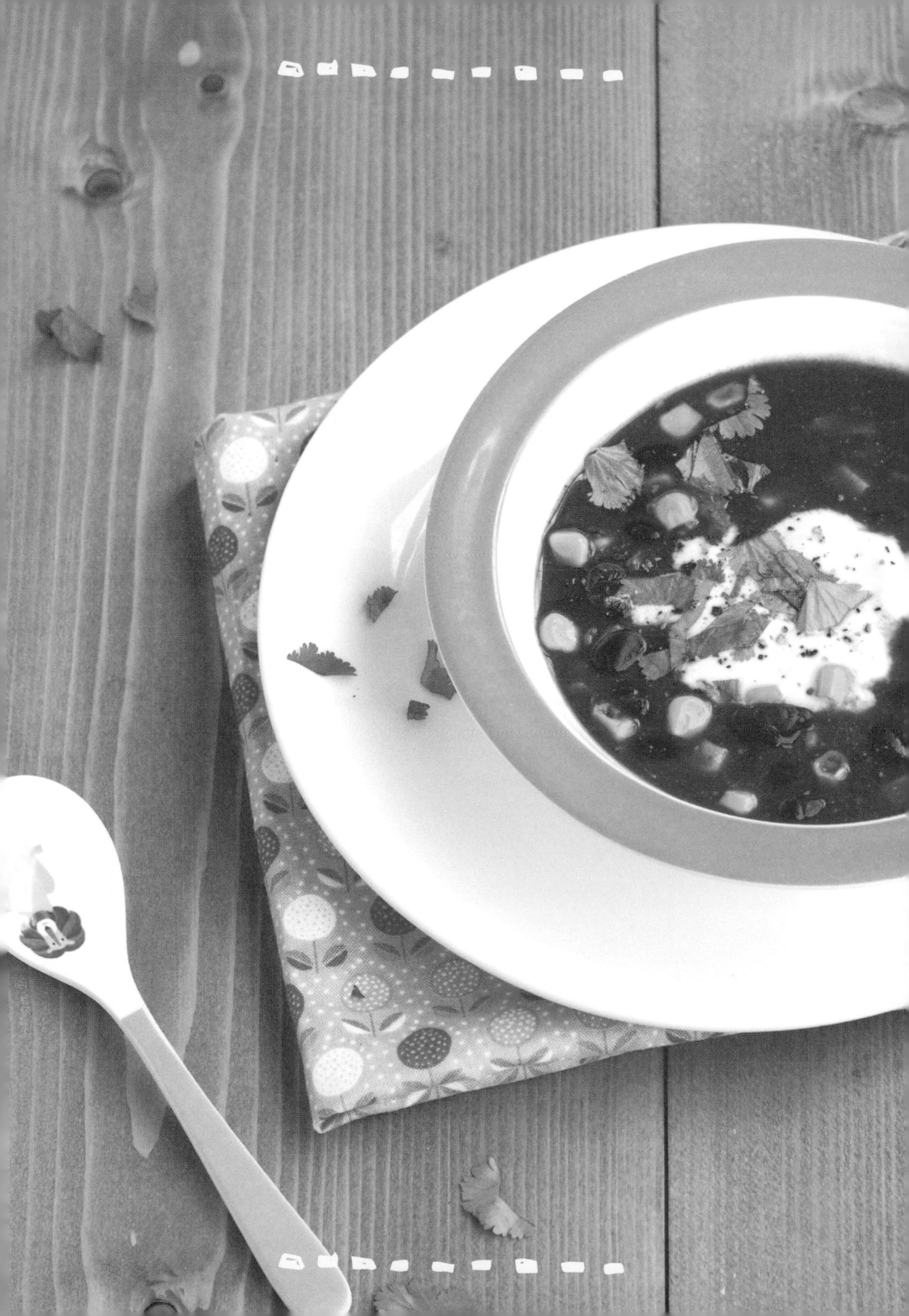

Butternut Squash & Coconut Soup

A deliciously creamy soup that will nourish your little one on the coldest, wettest days. This soup is so easy to make and will fill your kitchen with the most incredible smells.

Serves 2 adults and 2 children

1 butternut squash, peeled, deseeded and cut into chunks

3 red onions, peeled and quartered

1 whole bulb garlic (about 10 cloves)

olive oil, for roasting

400g full-fat coconut milk

1 litre water or homemade vegetable stock

¼ teaspoon ground cumin

1 teaspoon turmeric

1 teaspoon smoked paprika

8 cardamon pods, seeds only

1 sprig fresh rosemary, leaves picked and chopped

4 tablespoons Greek yogurt

Preheat oven to 180°C/350°F/gas 4.

Place the chunks of squash on a baking tray and add the onions and garlic. I leave the skins on the garlic cloves when roasting as it helps to keep the flavour in and stops it going dry. Drizzle the vegetables with a little olive oil and then roast for about 30 minutes, until the butternut squash is soft enough to stick a knife through.

When the vegetables are cooked, squeeze the garlic cloves out of their skins and then put everything (except the skins) into a large pot. Add all of the remaining ingredients, except the yogurt, to the pot and heat slowly until piping hot.

Remove from the heat and, using a stick blender, blend everything until smooth. You are looking for a consistency that can be sucked up through a straw. If you need to add more water, do so 60ml at a time. Stir in the Greek yogurt until fully combined.

Serve with some brown bread or in a sippy cup.

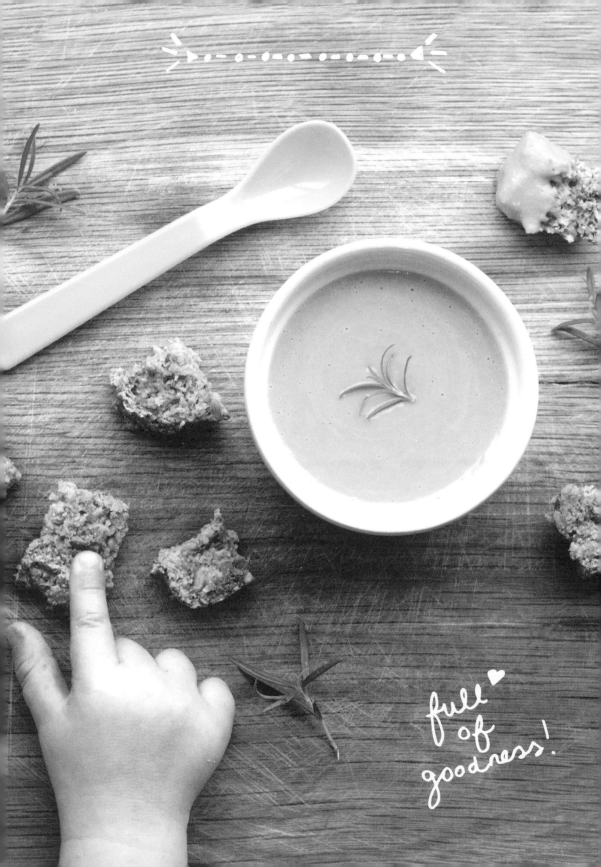

full of goodness!

Pull & Share
White Bread Rolls

I have my mother to thank for saving my sanity in my quest to make my own bread. A little extra egg, milk and double proving made all the difference and the result tastes delicious, is simple to make and looks amazing. Use this bread for baby sambos, burger buns and, best of all, for dipping into soup.

Makes 20 baby rolls

1 tbsp (20g): 12.1g free sugar
(20 servings) 0.6g each

150ml cold milk

150ml warm water

7g fast-acting dried yeast

1 tablespoon maple syrup

2 eggs

550g plain flour

1 egg yolk, beaten, for egg wash

Mix milk and water in a jug. It should be just warm, as if it's too hot it will kill the yeast. Add the yeast and maple syrup and give it a good stir. Leave aside in a warm place for about 10 minutes until it starts to become foamy. Then whisk in the eggs.

Sieve the flour into a large bowl and make a well in the middle. Add the wet mixture to the flour and stir until it starts to come together into a ball.

Turn the dough out onto a well-floured surface and knead for 10 minutes. (You can also use a food mixer if it has a dough hook.) The dough should become smoother and more stretchy by the end of this time. Put the dough into a floured bowl and cover with a tea towel. Keep in a warm place for about an hour or until it has roughly doubled in sized.

When proved, cut into 20 equal pieces and then roll into little dough balls using your hands. Arrange on a floured baking tray in a circle and press gently together to close any gaps. Cover and leave to prove a second time for about 45 minutes. The balls should have expanded again.

Meanwhile, preheat the oven to 200°C/400°F/gas 6. When the dough balls have proved, brush them with a little beaten egg yolk and bake for about 20 minutes or until golden on top. You may need to turn the tray around in the oven after about 15 minutes to ensure they cook evenly. Cool fully on a wire rack before serving.

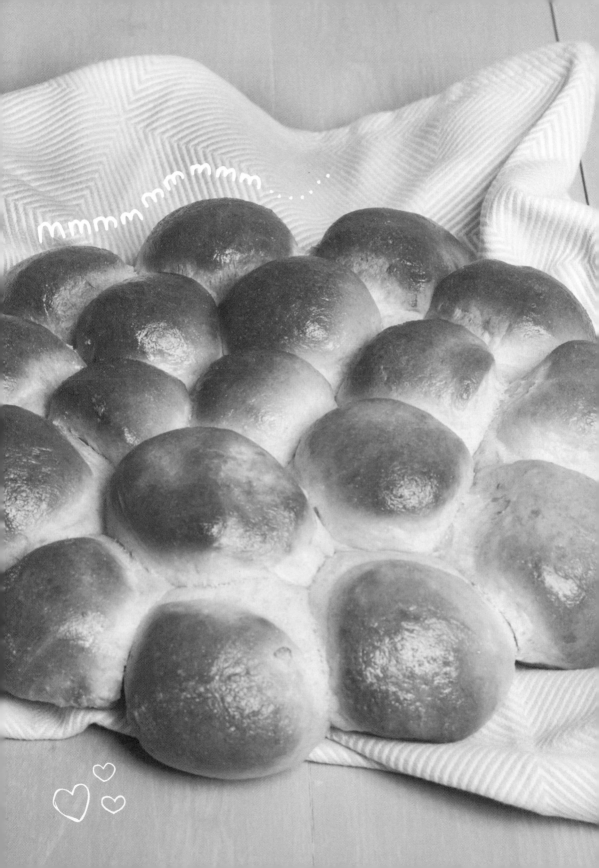

Granny's 10-Minute
Brown Bread

My mother, aka the granny in 'Granny's 10-Minute Brown Bread', gave me this recipe to share as it is one of my kids' favourites. It is also one of the quickest and easiest recipes in this book. You can change around the ingredients to suit your own tastes, and it is the perfect bread to help babies eat soup. Just dip some squares of bread into the soup for 30 seconds, then remove and let them get to work feeding themselves! It is also lovely with chia jam (see page 193).

Makes 1lb loaf

40g sunflower seeds

40g pumpkin seeds

180g stoneground wholemeal flour

150g oats

4 tablespoons chia seeds

4 tablespoons goji berries, chopped (optional)

1 teaspoon bicarbonate of soda

400ml buttermilk

Preheat oven to 200°C/400°F/gas 6.

First add the sunflower and pumpkin seeds to a pestle and mortar and grind down slightly so that they are still rough but not whole. This makes it easier for little mouths to eat.

Then place all the dry ingredients into a large mixing bowl and stir to combine. Make a well in the middle and pour in the buttermilk. Stir until the entire mixture is covered in the liquid.

Line a loaf tin with parchment paper, then pour the mixture in and spread evenly. I tap the bottom of the tin a few times on the counter to release any air bubbles.

Bake in the oven for 50 minutes. If you stick a skewer into the centre, it should come out clean.

Wrap the bread in a clean tea towel and leave to cool. This is important for little ones as it prevents the crust from going too hard.

Savoury Scones with Ham & Cheese

What better way to eat ham and cheese than mixed into a delicious brown scone! The smell of these cooking alone will bring back all kinds of childhood memories for grown-ups. Serve with a little unsalted butter and you have a perfect lunch for little ones.

Makes 16 scones (using 5cm cutter)

125g plain flour

125g stoneground wholemeal flour

2 teaspoons baking powder

60g unsalted butter

sprig rosemary, leaves picked and chopped

small bunch chives, finely chopped

50g grated cheddar cheese

200g fresh cooked ham, finely diced

150ml milk

1 free-range egg

Preheat oven to 200°C/400°F/gas 6.

In a large bowl, add the flours and baking powder. Using your fingers, rub in the butter until the mixture starts to resemble rough breadcrumbs.

Make a well in the centre of the flour mixture, then add the rosemary, chives, cheddar cheese and ham.

In a separate jug, whisk the milk and egg and pour into the flour. Stir until a dough begins to form, then tip out onto a well-floured surface.

Roll the dough out until it is about 3cm thick. Cut scones out with a small round cookie cutter or a glass. Remember, they are for little hands so smaller is better.

Transfer to a baking tray lined with parchment paper and bake for about 25 minutes until they are golden.

Serve with a little unsalted butter.

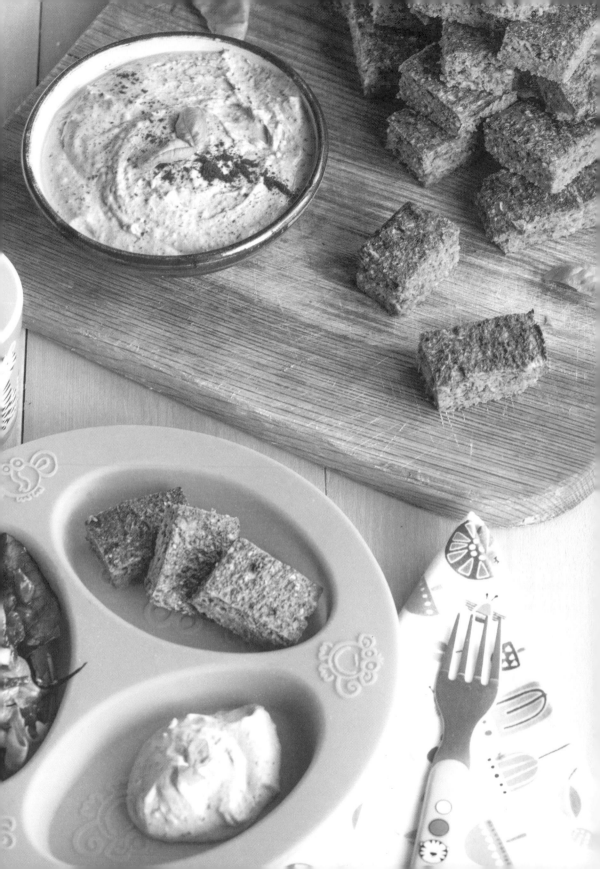

Veggie Bread

Bread is a staple food in most Irish households and my kids would live on the stuff if we let them. This bread, however, is one that I wouldn't mind if they ate every day, as it is jam-packed with good, nourishing ingredients. It is delicious eaten with hummus (see pages 196–7) and tastes so yummy they'll never guess it's so good for them!

Serves 2 adults and 2 children

70g spinach

180g cauliflower, roughly chopped

180g broccoli, roughly chopped

2 small carrots, roughly chopped

small bunch parsley

200g spelt flour

1 teaspoon bicarbonate of soda

3 eggs

ground pepper, to season

Preheat oven to 180°C/350°F/gas 4.

Add the spinach, cauliflower, broccoli, carrot and parsley to a food processor and pulse until they resemble breadcrumbs. (You may have to do this in batches if you have a small food processor.)

Put the blitzed vegetables into a large bowl, then add the flour, bicarbonate of soda, eggs and pepper and stir until totally combined.

Turn onto a 35 x 23cm baking tin lined with parchment paper and flatten with the back of a spoon. Bake for about 25 minutes or until it has set.

Allow it to cool fully, then flip over and peel off the paper. Cut into fingers.

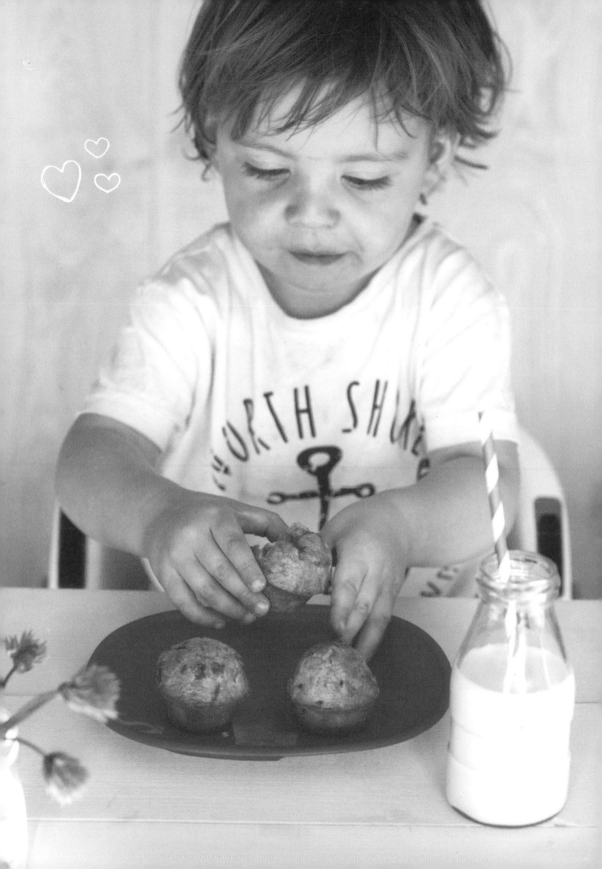

Courgette & Cheese
Baby Muffins

Deliciously healthy lunchtime muffins that are a real kid-pleaser. I've been making these for Oscar since he was just six months old and they remain one of his favourites. Make a big batch and keep them in the freezer for those days you're out and about and need a nourishing snack in a hurry.

Makes 24 mini-muffins

320g plain flour

3 teaspoons baking powder

250ml whole milk

2 eggs

60ml rapeseed oil

1 medium courgette, grated

50g grated cheddar cheese

sprig fresh rosemary, leaves picked and chopped

black pepper, to season

1 teaspoon Dijon mustard

Preheat oven to 200°C/400°F/gas 6.

Sieve flour and baking powder into a large mixing bowl.

In a jug, whisk together the milk, eggs and rapeseed oil.

Make a well in the centre of the flour and slowly whisk in the wet mixture until it forms a smooth batter.

Squeeze the grated courgette to remove some of the liquid before adding to the bowl along with the cheddar cheese, rosemary, pepper and mustard. Give everything a good stir.

Spoon the mixture into an oiled mini-muffin tin or into muffin cases. Bake for 25 minutes until the muffins have risen and are golden brown – when you stick a toothpick into them it should come out clean.

Serve warm or cold.

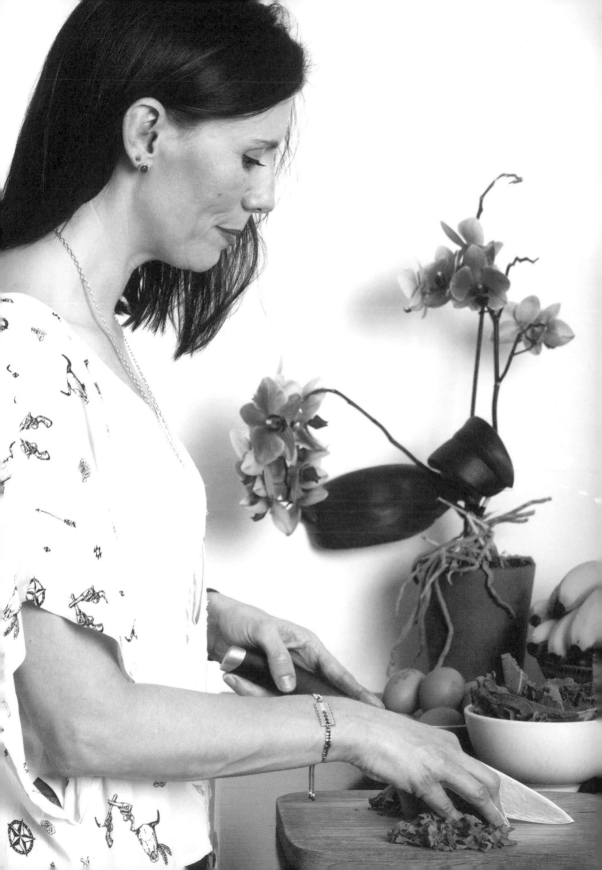

Kale & Cheese
Muffins

These probably won't win any prizes for good looks but they are so good for you that it really doesn't matter. I have brought these to the zoo and on picnics and they are so handy for those busy days when you want something nourishing for your baby but don't fancy cooking up a storm.

Makes 24 mini-muffins

150g plain flour
1 teaspoon baking powder
50g kale
125ml milk
1 egg
50g goat's cheese

Preheat oven to 200°C/400°F/gas 6.

Sieve the flour and baking powder into a large bowl.

Add the kale and milk to a blender and blend until no bits of kale are showing – it should resemble bright-green milk! Add the egg and pulse a few times more.

Make a well in the flour and pour the liquid slowly into it, making sure to stir to prevent lumps. Keep going until all of the milk has been added and you're left with a batter.

Break up the goat's cheese and fold into the mixture, then pour into muffin cases and bake for 25–30 minutes or until the muffins are golden and a toothpick comes out clean.

Serve warm or cold.

Sweet Potato
Super Muffins

Nutritious and perfect for little tummies at lunch time, these fragrant muffins are so easy to make and also freeze really well – ideal for busy days when you need something yummy quickly!

Makes 24 mini-muffins

320g plain flour

3 teaspoons baking powder

250ml milk

2 eggs

60ml rapeseed oil

250g cooked sweet potato

6 cloves garlic, roasted

sprig fresh rosemary, leaves picked and chopped

Preheat oven to 200°C/400°F/gas 6.

Sieve flour and baking powder into a large mixing bowl.

In a jug, whisk together the milk, eggs and rapeseed oil. Make a well in the centre of the flour and slowly whisk in the wet mixture until it forms a smooth batter.

Add the sweet potato and roasted garlic to a blender and blend until smooth and creamy. Fold into the muffin batter along with the rosemary.

Spoon the mixture into an oiled mini-muffin tin and bake for 25 minutes. The muffins should be golden on top and a toothpick should come out clean.

Serve warm or cold.

Tuna and Quinoa Baby Bites

These little bites are yummy and so healthy for little weaning babies. I use line-caught tuna because it has such a meaty texture and it goes really well with veggies and quinoa. The bites freeze really well and make a wholesome lunch for babies and kids of all ages.

Makes 24 mini-muffins

625ml water

100g uncooked quinoa

2 tablespoons olive oil

140g broccoli, finely chopped

1 white onion, finely chopped

2 cloves garlic, crushed

60g baby leaf spinach, finely chopped

300g tinned tuna

¼ teaspoon black pepper

1 lemon, juice only

2 sprigs fresh parsley

1 teaspoon Dijon mustard

6 eggs

3 tablespoons natural yogurt

Bring the water to the boil, then add the quinoa, stir and turn the heat down to a simmer. Cover the pot and cook for 20 minutes or until the water has been absorbed completely and the quinoa is light and fluffy.

Heat the olive oil in a saucepan and fry the broccoli, onion and garlic until the onion starts to turn translucent.

Put the quinoa, fried vegetables, spinach and tuna into a large bowl. Season with a little pepper then squeeze in the lemon juice.

Add the parsley and Dijon mustard to a jug, crack in the eggs and yogurt, then whisk it all up until the eggs have become light and bubbly. Pour into the quinoa mixture and stir really well.

Spoon the mixture into a mini-muffin tin lined with mini-muffin cases and bake for 30 minutes or until the mixture has fully set.

Serve warm.

Healthy Baked Beans

Beans – one of the most popular convenience foods in Ireland and the UK. They are such a handy food to give to kids. This recipe is true to the traditional qualities of baked beans – saucy, sweet and really filling – yet these contain no refined sugar or salt and I think they're nicer than the processed store-bought kind. Make a big batch and freeze in little portions for your own homemade convenience food.

Makes about 1,200g

rapeseed oil, for frying

1 large onion, chopped

2 cloves garlic, crushed

2 tablespoons unsalted tomato purée

400g tinned tomatoes

400ml water (in two lots of 200ml)

4 Medjool dates

800g tinned unsalted butter beans

1 teaspoon smoked paprika

2 teaspoons apple cider vinegar

1 teaspoon tamarind paste or lime juice

Preheat oven to 160°C/325°F/gas 3.

Heat the oil in a frying pan and gently fry the onion over a medium heat until golden. Add the garlic and cook for a further 2–3 minutes until soft but not browned. Then add the tomato purée, tinned tomatoes and 200ml of water and stir well.

Transfer this mixture to a blender, add the Medjool dates and purée until completely smooth. (If you don't have a high-speed blender you might want to soak your dates in warm water for about an hour beforehand.)

Pour the mixture into a deep oven dish and add the remaining ingredients. Give it all a good stir to completely combine.

Bake in the oven for about 60 minutes. Stir in the other 200ml of water and then bake for another 60 minutes (2 hours in total).

Remove from the oven and leave to cool slightly before serving. If the sauce is a little thick you can add more water.

Serve with homemade brown-bread soldiers.

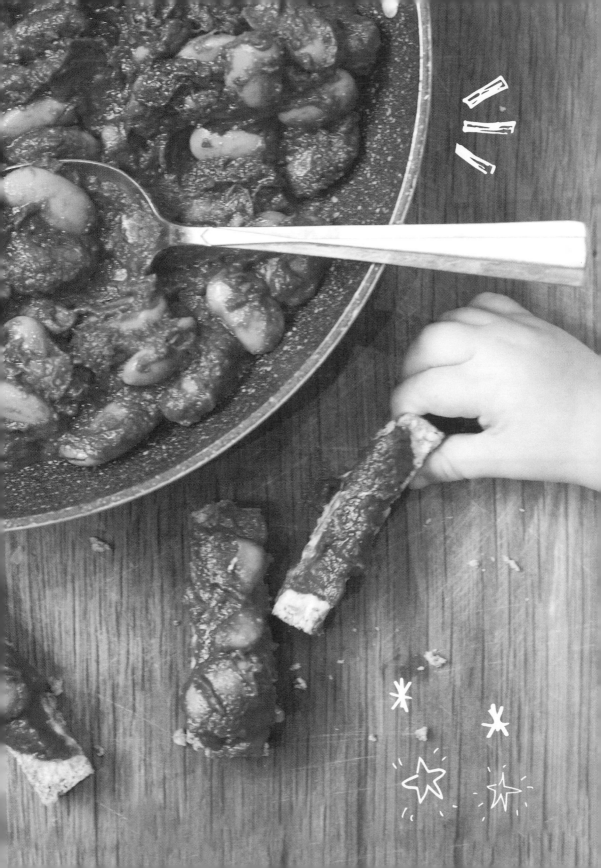

Super Baby Frittatas
with Greens

These are called 'super baby frittatas' because of the amazing ingredients used. Spinach is one of my favourite vegetables and is an amazing source of iron, which little weaning babies need. It is also packed with a multitude of other vitamins and minerals.

Makes 24 mini-frittatas

olive oil, for frying

1 medium onion, chopped

2 cloves garlic, crushed

80g green beans, finely chopped

80g peas

30g spinach, roughly chopped

4 eggs

2 tablespoons milk

½ teaspoon Dijon mustard

10 basil leaves, finely chopped

Preheat oven to 180°C/350°F/gas 4.

Heat some oil in a pan and gently fry the onion for about 5 minutes over a medium heat. Add the garlic, green beans and peas and cook for 3–5 minutes, until the beans become soft. Then add the spinach and stir until it starts to wilt. Remove the pan from the heat and set aside.

In a large bowl, beat the eggs, milk and mustard and then add the contents of the pan to the bowl, along with the basil.

Add the mixture to a well-oiled mini-muffin tin, making sure each cup is filled to the top.

Bake for 20 minutes or until the frittatas are golden brown on top.

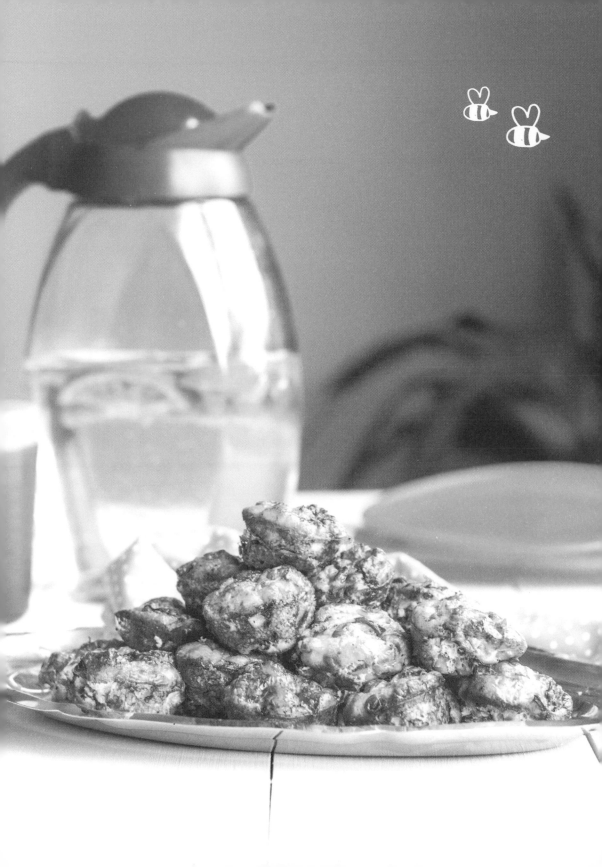

Rainbow Fritters
with Carrot, Beetroot and Peas

The combination of vegetables just looks so colourful – my kids devour these straight out of the oven. They make a great lunchtime snack and are so good for you and your little ones, as they are packed with great ingredients.

Makes 12

100g raw beetroot, peeled and grated

70g carrot, grated

2 tablespoons flour

80g peas

2 eggs

pinch black pepper

1 tablespoon rapeseed oil

Preheat oven to 190°C/375°F/gas 5.

Add all of the ingredients to a large bowl and mix well until fully combined.

Shape into patties and place on a baking sheet lined with parchment paper.

Lightly brush the tops of each patty with a little oil, then bake for 12 minutes. Take out of the oven and flip over. Lightly brush the top of the unbaked side with oil then bake for another 12 minutes or until golden.

Serve with a little Baby Ketchup (page 203) or Spinach & Garlic Creamy Dip (page 202).

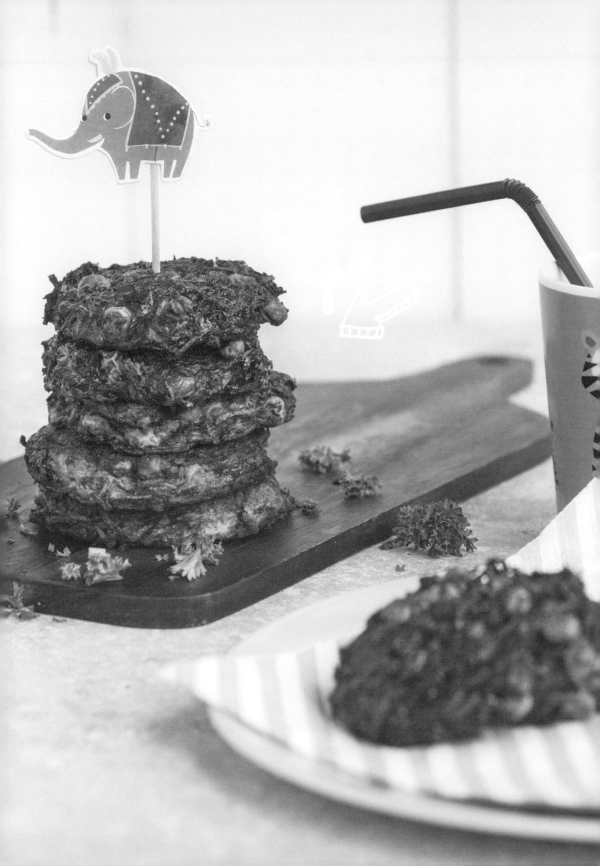

Butternut Squash
Frittatas

Frittatas are such a simple dish and these ones are just fab! They are ideal for starting off weaning as they are soft and can be filled with so many nutritious ingredients. They're handy for days when you're out and about, so make a big batch and stock up your freezer.

Makes 24 mini-frittatas

1 tablespoon rapeseed oil or olive oil

3 shallots or 1 medium-sized onion, finely chopped

2 cloves garlic, crushed

4 eggs

250ml milk

100g goat's cheese

¼ teaspoon nutmeg

pinch black pepper

200g roasted butternut squash

Preheat oven to 180°C/350°F/gas 4.

Heat the oil in a frying pan and add the shallots. Fry, stirring constantly, for about 5 minutes before adding the garlic and cooking for a further 2–3 minutes. This step is important, as the garlic and shallots can be quite strong for little tastebuds.

In a bowl, whisk the eggs and milk together until light and bubbly, then crumble in the cheese and sprinkle in the nutmeg and pepper.

Chop the butternut squash into little cubes and then add to the egg mixture. Finally, add the fried shallot and garlic and stir well until fully combined.

Brush a mini-muffin tin with some extra oil and then spoon the mixture in evenly.

Bake for about 15 minutes until the frittatas have fully set.

Allow to cool before serving.

Sweetcorn Fritters

I wasn't sure whether to call these fritters or pancakes, as they use a regular pancake batter but taste more like a delicious fritter. It took a while for my little dude to love corn, and at first he would pick the corn pieces out bit by bit, but eventually hunger got the better of him and now they're one of his favourite foods!

Makes 16

150g plain flour

2 teaspoons baking powder

250ml milk

1 organic egg

2 tablespoons melted unsalted butter

2 spring onions, finely chopped

80g sweetcorn

50g cheddar cheese, grated

¼ teaspoon ground nutmeg

¼ teaspoon paprika

butter or rapeseed oil, for frying

Sieve the flour and baking powder into a large bowl.

In a separate bowl, mix together the milk, egg and melted unsalted butter.

Make a well in the flour and slowly whisk in the liquid mixture until completely combined. Add the spring onions, sweetcorn, cheese and spices to the batter, making sure to mix well.

Heat a large frying pan over a medium heat. For each batch of pancakes, melt about 1 teaspoon of unsalted butter or rapeseed oil.

Spoon 2–3 tablespoons of batter into the pan for each fritter. Cook until you see bubbles forming (about 1–2 minutes). Flip over and cook the other side. Transfer fritters to a plate and leave in a warm oven while you cook the next batch.

Serve warm.

Butternut Squash
Pancakes

Butternut squash not only tastes great, it is also one of the most nutritious vegetables you can eat. It contains significant amounts of fibre, is rich in vitamins, minerals and antioxidants and, if that isn't enough, it's really filling. The combination of butternut squash, goat's cheese and rosemary with pancake batter may sound a bit crazy but it really works and is a delicious snack for your baby.

Makes 24 pancakes

150g plain flour

2 teaspoons baking powder

250ml milk

1 egg

2 tablespoons melted unsalted butter

200g roasted butternut squash, puréed

3 tablespoons goat's cheese

small sprig fresh rosemary, leaves picked and chopped

rapeseed oil, for frying

Sieve flour and baking powder into a large bowl.

In a separate bowl, mix the milk, egg and melted unsalted butter.

Make a well in the flour and slowly whisk in the liquid mixture until completely combined. Fold the butternut squash purée into the batter and then crumble in the goat's cheese and add the rosemary.

Heat a large frying pan over a medium heat. For each batch of pancakes, use about 1 teaspoon rapeseed oil.

Spoon 2–3 tablespoons of batter into the pan. Cook until you see bubbles forming (about 1–2 minutes). Flip over and cook the other side.

Serve warm or cold.

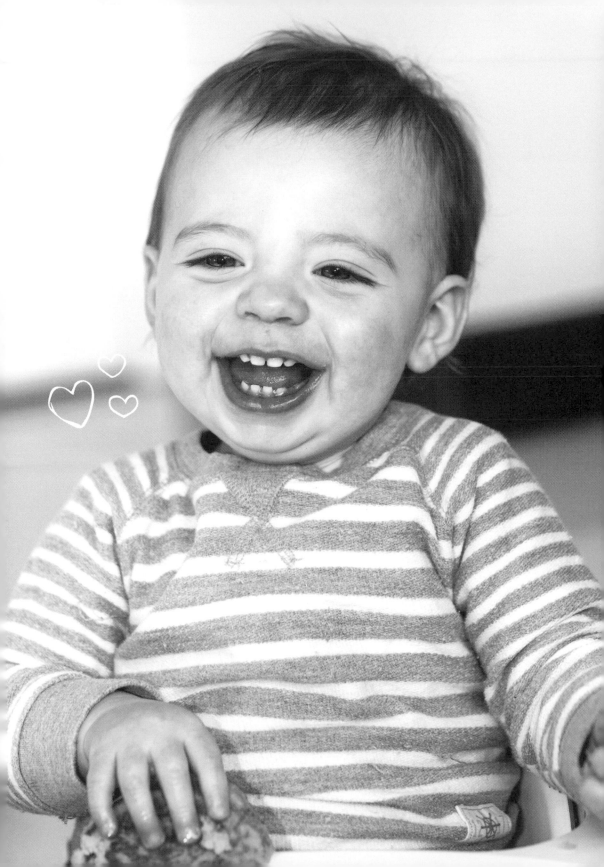

Cheesy Cauliflower
Baby Bites

The only problem with these little bites is stopping the grown-ups from eating them before the baby gets a chance. They are a great way to get little ones to eat cauliflower. I use just a little cheddar cheese but you can substitute goat's cheese if you like.

Makes 12

150g cauliflower, roughly chopped

50g onion, finely chopped

small bunch parsley

60g breadcrumbs

50g cheddar cheese, grated

1 tablespoon olive oil

1 egg, beaten

Preheat oven to 180ºC/350ºF/gas 4.

Add the cauliflower, onion and parsley to a food processor. Pulse until it's the texture of breadcrumbs, then pour into a large bowl.

Add the remaining ingredients and stir until completely mixed.

Shape into little rolls and place onto a lightly oiled baking tray. Bake for 12 minutes, then remove from the oven, flip over and bake for a further 12 minutes or until golden on both sides.

Cool before serving.

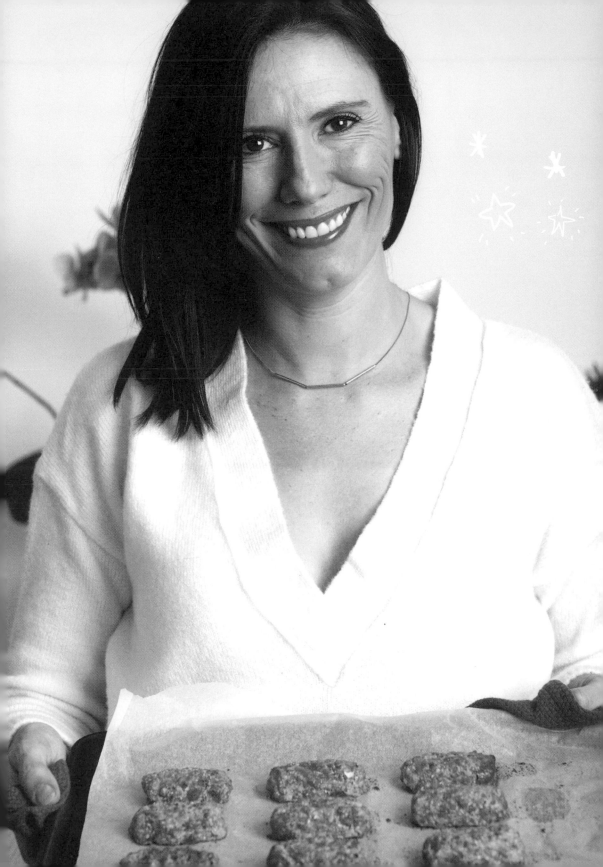

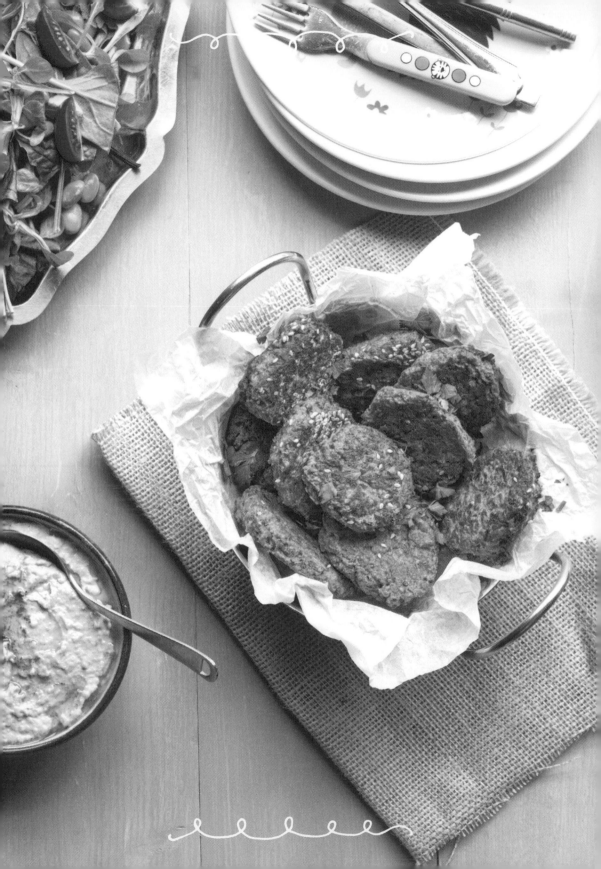

Falafel

Falafel are a traditional Middle Eastern street food made by combining chickpeas with spices, egg and a little flour. They are easy and quick to make, are pretty cheap and taste delicious, especially when paired with hummus and a baby salad. A satisfying, healthy fast food for all the family.

Makes 12

2 shallots, finely chopped

2 cloves garlic, crushed

400g tinned chickpeas

small bunch parsley, finely chopped

2 teaspoons ground coriander

2 teaspoons ground cumin

1 egg, beaten

2 tablespoons flour

rapeseed oil, for frying

Heat a drizzle of rapeseed oil in a pan, then add the shallots and fry gently. They will start to caramelise after about 6 minutes. Add the garlic and fry for a further 2–3 minutes until the garlic is fragrant, then remove from the heat and set aside.

In a large bowl, add the chickpeas and mash with a fork until smooth and creamy. Add the parsley, coriander and cumin. Next, fold the egg into the mixture with the flour. Finally, add the onion and garlic and give everything a good stir.

Divide the mixture into 12 little patties. Heat 3–4 tablespoons of rapeseed oil in a frying pan until really hot then drop the falafel in and fry on both sides until golden.

Serve with hummus (see pages 196–7) and a baby salad of chopped soft lettuce leaves, quartered tomatoes and finely chopped spring onion.

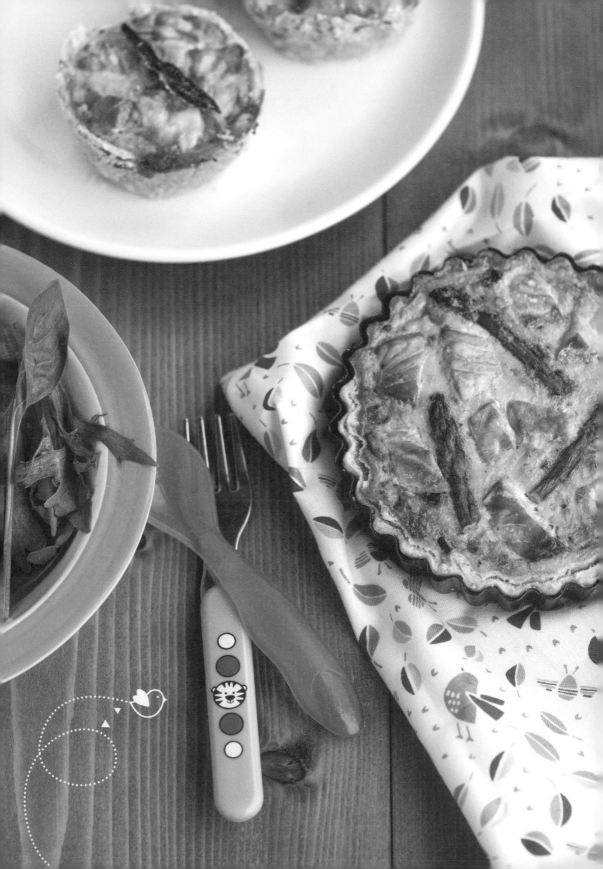

Baby Quiche with Salmon and Asparagus

Salmon is a wonderful food to feed your little one. It is so nutritious and is an excellent source of vitamins and minerals, but more importantly, it's a rich source of omega-3, which is known as 'brain food'.

Makes 12 baby quiches

For the pastry

150g plain flour

80g butter

2–3 tablespoons water

For the filling

2 tablespoons rapeseed oil

1 medium-sized onion, finely chopped

1 large clove garlic, crushed

100g courgette, finely chopped

6 asparagus stems, finely chopped (tips reserved for decoration)

6 eggs

2 tablespoons natural yogurt (optional)

sprinkle of pepper, to season

250g salmon fillet, cut into small cubes

Preheat oven to 200°C/400°F/gas 6.

To make the pastry, sieve the flour into a bowl and, using your fingers, work the butter in until the flour starts to resemble fine breadcrumbs. Add the water a tablespoon at a time until the pastry comes together. Wrap in cling film and refrigerate for about 30 minutes.

Place the pastry onto a lightly floured surface and roll until it measures about half a centimetre deep. Then cut out 12 circles to fit a standard muffin tin. Lightly butter a muffin tin and line each cup with a pastry case, then place in the fridge while you get on with the filling.

To make the filling, gently heat the rapeseed oil over a medium heat and fry the onion until it starts to turn soft. Then add the garlic and cook for another few minutes. Add the chopped courgette and asparagus stems to the pan and cook for about 3–4 minutes, until the courgette softens. Remove from the pan and leave aside.

In a bowl, whisk the eggs, yogurt and pepper until light and bubbly.

Remove the pastry from the fridge. Divide the vegetable mix between the pastry cases, add a few pieces of salmon to each one, then finally fill with the egg mixture. Chop the asparagus tips in half and then decorate each quiche with one.

Bake for 25 minutes or until the pastry is golden and the egg has fully set. Remove and cool before serving.

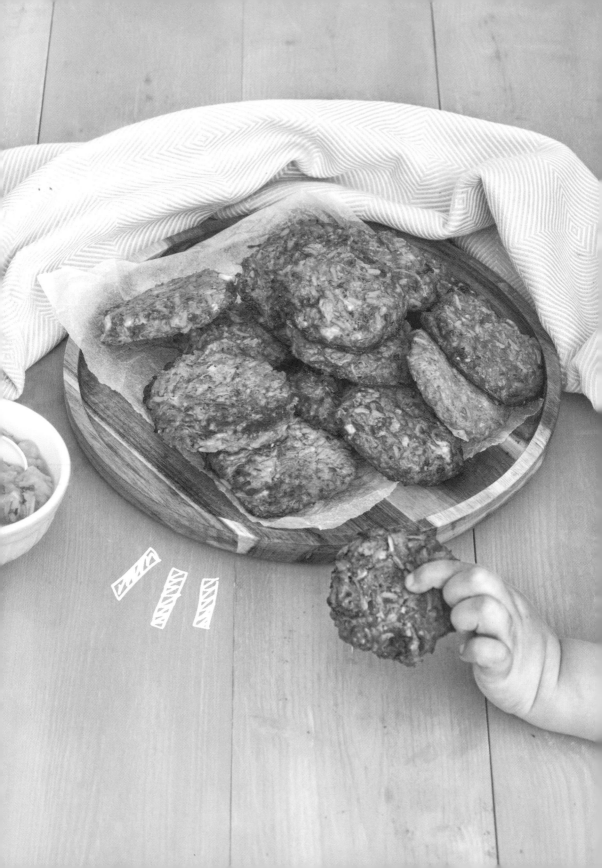

Tuna & Avocado Bhajis
with Mango Salsa

This recipe started off as tuna and avocado bites, but they didn't go according to plan so I added a little spice to make them more flavoursome. The result was an amazing mixture of flavours that tasted more like an Indian bhaji. My nine-year-old, who detests tuna, didn't even realise he was eating it until I told him afterwards. I serve these with a delicious mango salsa.

Makes 24 mini-bhajis

For the bhajis

110g cooked brown rice

1 ripe avocado, chopped

½ lemon, juice only

200g tin tuna, drained

small bunch coriander, finely chopped

100g carrot, grated

100g broccoli, finely chopped

1 teaspoon ground cumin

1 teaspoon turmeric

1 teaspoon paprika

150g plain flour

250ml water

3 tablespoons rapeseed oil

For the mango salsa

½ mango, finely chopped

½ sweet red onion, finely chopped

small bunch coriander, finely chopped

½ lime, juice only

Preheat oven to 200°C/400°F/gas 6.

Place all of the bhaji ingredients, except for the flour, water and oil, in a large bowl. Sprinkle the flour over the mixture and stir until the vegetables and fish are completely coated.

Make a well in the centre of the mix, then slowly pour in the water and oil, stirring as you do. Keep going until all the liquid is gone and the mixture has turned into a thick batter.

Spoon heaped tablespoons of the batter onto a tray lined with parchment paper, then shape with the back of a spoon into little patties.

Bake for 25–30 minutes until the bhajis turn golden brown and are completely set.

Meanwhile, make the mango salsa. Place the mango, onion and coriander in a bowl, squeeze over the lime juice and give it a good mix.

When the bhajis are cooled and ready to eat, serve with a little salsa on each one.

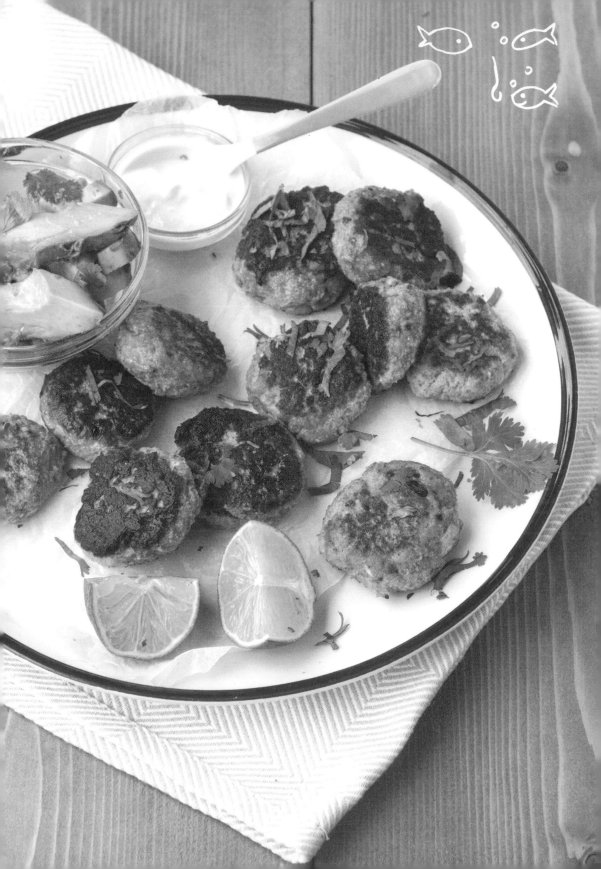

Salmon Fishy Cakes with Avocado & Yogurt and Lime Dressing

These little fish cakes are the perfect way to introduce your baby to salmon. They are soft, full of nutritious goodness and shaped into small, perfectly sized burgers that your little one will just love. They freeze really well and defrost quickly because of their size, so make a double or triple batch to have healthy lunches ready for busy days.

Makes 24 mini-fishcakes

1 tsp (5g): 3g free sugar
(24 servings) 0.12g each

For the fishcakes

250g raw salmon fillet, roughly chopped

1 small onion, roughly chopped

1 egg

60g breadcrumbs

black pepper, to season

½ teaspoon paprika

2 tablespoons rapeseed oil, for frying

For the dressing

4 tablespoons Greek yogurt

1 teaspoon maple syrup

½ lime, juice only

1 avocado, chopped, to serve

Add the salmon and onion to a food processor and process until it becomes a paste. Add in the egg, breadcrumbs, pepper and paprika and mix well.

Spoon a heaped tablespoon of the mixture at a time into your hand and shape into small baby-sized fishcakes.

Heat the oil on a frying pan and gently fry both sides of the cakes until golden and cooked through.

To make the dressing, place all the ingredients in a bowl and stir well.

Serve the fishcakes with dressing and chopped avocado on the side.

Baby-Friendly
Salmon Pâté

Salmon is an excellent source of vitamins, minerals and omega-3 and is a great first food to give your little ones. Eat this dish fresh to get the most from the nutritious ingredients.

Serves 1 adult and 1 child

200g fresh organic salmon

4 tablespoons natural yogurt

90g cream cheese

10 sprigs fresh parsley

4 cloves garlic, roasted

½ lemon, juice and zest

pinch black pepper

¼ teaspoon paprika

1 teaspoon Dijon mustard

Using a steamer, cook the salmon for about 15 minutes. Remove from the heat and leave aside to cool fully.

Once the salmon has cooled, add all of the ingredients to a food processor and blitz until completely smooth. Serve with flour tortillas (see page 143).

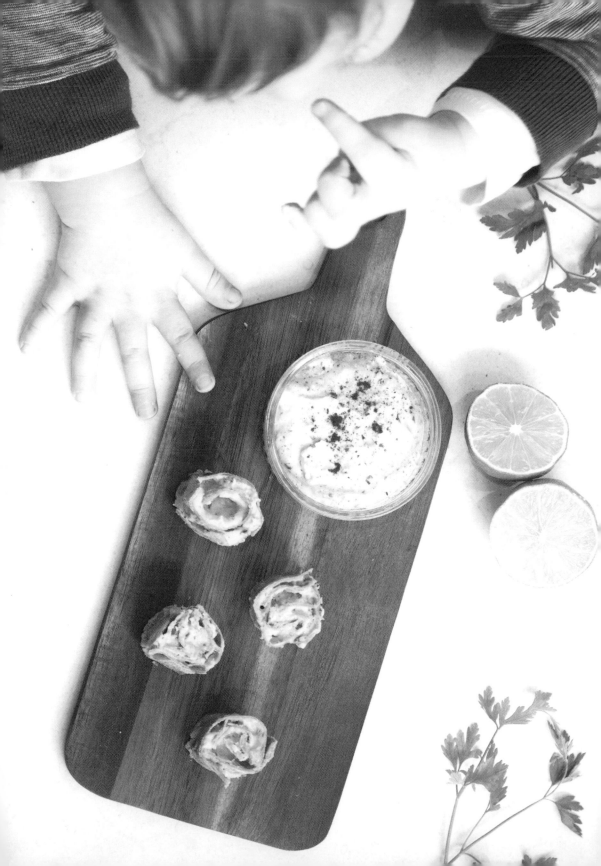

Beef Empanadas

On a lovely summer holiday in Spain we all got totally addicted to empanadas. They are a traditional Argentinian street food that can be eaten either warm or cold. I've made them with every concoction of fillings but these particular ones are our favourite so far. They are the ideal size for little hands to manage so are perfect for weaning.

Makes 24 mini-empanadas

For the pastry

300g plain flour

160g unsalted butter

2 medium eggs

4–6 tablespoons water

For the filling

rapeseed oil, for frying

1 medium red onion, finely diced

2 cloves garlic, crushed

1 red bell pepper, finely diced

200g lean minced beef

200g tinned chopped tomatoes

1 teaspoon paprika

½ teaspoon ground coriander

½ teaspoon ground cumin

¼ teaspoon mild chilli powder

1 egg, beaten, for egg wash

Preheat oven to 180°C/350°F/gas 4.

Sieve the flour into a bowl. Add the butter and 2 eggs and, using your fingers, rub them into the flour until it resembles fine breadcrumbs. Add the water 1 tablespoon at a time, using your hands to mix, until the pastry sticks together. Form into a ball, wrap in cling film and refrigerate for about an hour.

Heat the rapeseed oil in a frying pan over a medium heat and gently fry the onion for about 8 minutes until it starts to caramelise and turn sticky and sweet. Add the garlic and cook for a further 2–3 minutes. Then add the pepper and minced beef and stir well until the meat starts to brown.

Add the remaining ingredients for the filling to the pan, stir well and simmer for 20 minutes until the sauce starts to thicken. Remove from the heat.

Take the pastry from the fridge and roll it out on a floured surface until thin. Cut out roughly 16 circles.

Spoon 2 tablespoons of the filling into the centre of each pastry circle and then fold into a semicircle. Pinch the edges to make sure they are sealed, then place on an oiled baking sheet.

Brush each empanada with a little egg wash and then bake for 30 minutes or until golden brown. Serve warm or cool.

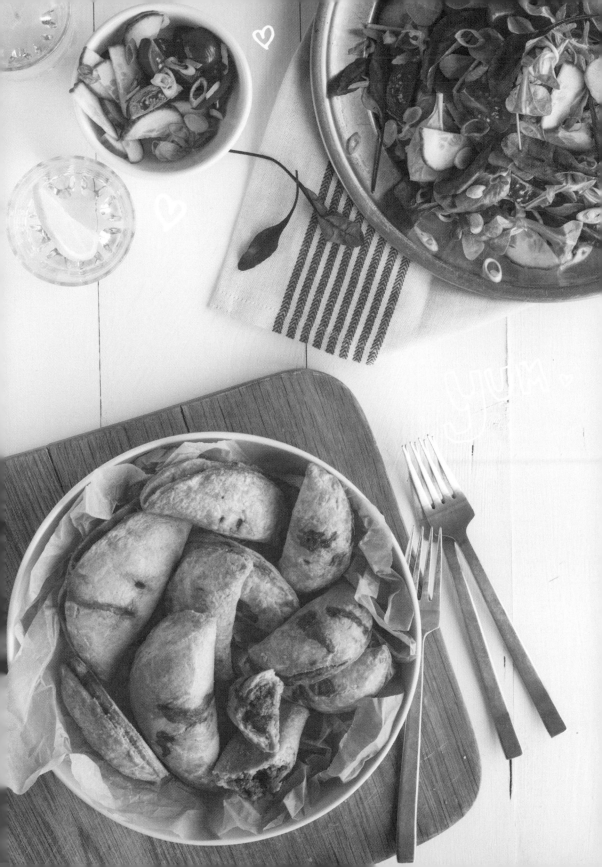

Spinach & Cream
Baby Pies

These delicate little pies are a brilliant way of getting your baby to eat more of the green stuff. Spinach provides lots of vitamins as well as extra fibre, calcium and many other minerals. The pies look so pretty when cooked and taste so good that your only problem will be getting everyone else in the house to keep their mitts off.

Makes 24 mini-pies

For the pastry

150g plain flour

80g unsalted butter

1 medium egg

3–4 tablespoons water

For the filling

3 shallots, finely chopped

rapeseed oil, for frying

2 cloves garlic, crushed

4 large handfuls baby spinach leaves, roughly chopped

4 tablespoons Parmesan cheese, grated

125ml cream

1 teaspoon Dijon mustard

black pepper, to season

1 egg, beaten, for egg wash

Preheat oven to 180°C/350°F/gas 4.

Sieve the flour into a bowl. Add the butter and egg and, using your fingers, rub into the flour until it resembles fine breadcrumbs. Add the water 1 tablespoon at a time, using your hands to mix until the pastry sticks together. Form into a ball, wrap in cling film and refrigerate for about an hour.

Gently fry the shallots in the rapeseed oil over a medium heat until they start to turn translucent. Add the garlic and cook for a further 2–3 minutes, making sure you don't let the garlic burn.

Add the spinach, cheese, cream, mustard and pepper to the pan. Stir well and cook for just 1 minute. The spinach should be slightly wilted but not cooked. Remove from the heat and leave aside.

Take the dough out of the fridge and, using a rolling pin, roll it out until it is about half a centimetre thick. Cut out 24 small discs and fit a disc into each cup of a lightly oiled mini-muffin tin.

Spoon a heaped teaspoon of the spinach cream mixture into each pie, then bake for 25 minutes until the pastry is golden.

Serve warm.

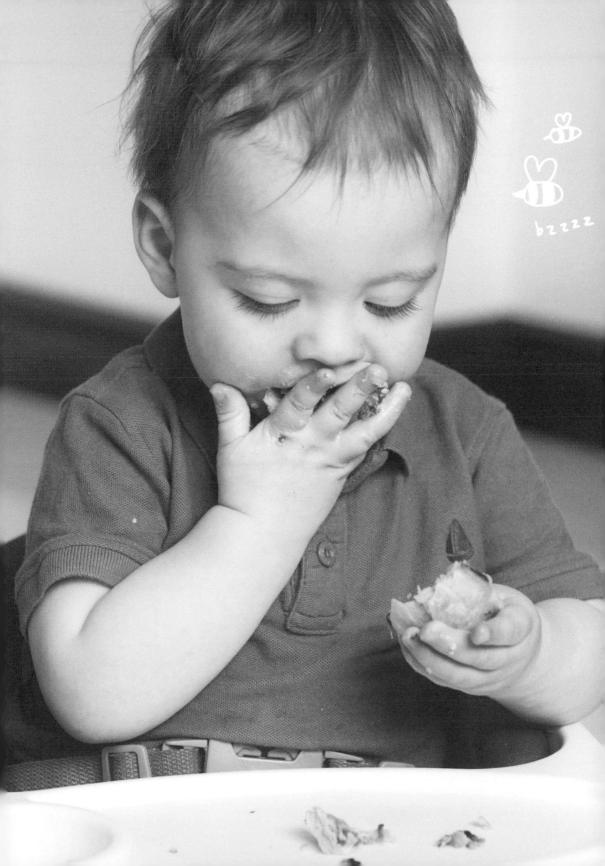

Stir-Fried Veg
with Panda Rice

I bought a rice maker online recently that moulds rice into the cutest little pandas. I make the eyes, ears and mouth for this from seaweed, although I've used kale too before and it worked just as well. This dish is easy to make and contains only simple ingredients, but sometimes that's all you need to make something delicious.

Serves 1 adult and 1 child

1 tsp (5g): 3g free sugar
(4 servings) 0.75g each

60g rice

½ teaspoon cider vinegar (or white vinegar)

25g broccoli, chopped into spears

50g courgette, chopped into spears

25g red pepper, chopped into spears

2 teaspoons olive oil

¼ teaspoon ground coriander

1 tablespoon tahini

1 teaspoon maple syrup

1 teaspoon lime juice

1 sprig fresh coriander, finely chopped

Add the rice to a saucepan along with 160ml water. Bring to the boil, then cover with a lid and turn off the heat, allowing the rice to steam cook. This should take about 10 minutes. Leave the lid on – don't remove until you are ready to serve.

Steam the broccoli until soft. While it is cooking, heat the oil in a frying pan and gently fry the other vegetables until soft too.

Add the broccoli to the pan along with the remaining ingredients, except for the fresh coriander, and stir well until the vegetables are fully coated.

Serve the vegetables with the cooked rice and sprinkle with fresh coriander.

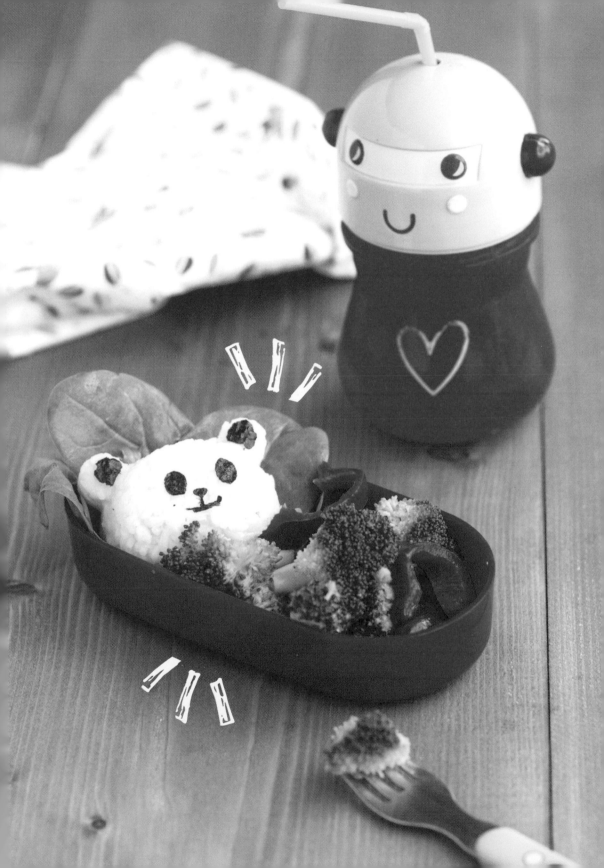

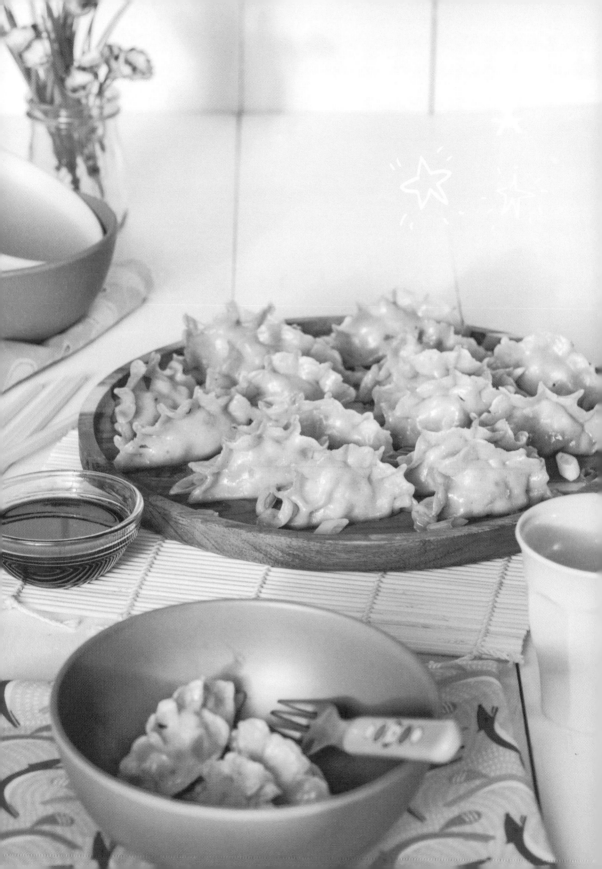

Gyoza Dumplings
with Pork, Spinach and Peas

Gyoza dumplings originate from Japan – however, they are also known as potstickers or dumplings in China and are a common food eaten during Chinese New Year. You can buy the dough pre-made but, as it contains preservatives, I prefer to make my own. Don't be alarmed at the thought of it, though. It is very easy and contains just two ingredients – flour and water! And your little ones will love eating veggies and meat all wrapped up in a delicious casing.

Makes 20 dumplings

For the dough

175g plain flour

120ml boiling water

For the filling

3 tablespoons sesame oil, plus extra for frying

15g ginger root, thinly sliced

3 shallots, finely chopped

300g minced pork

50g baby spinach leaves, roughly chopped

80g peas

black pepper, to taste

120ml boiling water, to cook

To make the pastry, sieve the flour into a bowl and make a well in the middle. Add the boiling water and, using a spatula, stir until it becomes a dough. You may need a little extra water – just add one tablespoon at a time.

Once dough is cool enough to touch, knead for about 5 minutes.

Cut the dough into 2 parts and roll into long sausage shapes. Then slice each sausage into 10 pieces. It is much easier to roll out these smaller pieces.

Using a rolling pin, on a well-floured surface, roll each piece of dough into a thin circle. Layer on top of each other and refrigerate until you are ready to add the filling.

Heat the sesame oil in a pan over a medium heat and add the ginger and chopped shallots. Fry until the shallots become translucent (about 2–3 minutes) then add the minced pork and fry until it's brown and cooked through. Add the spinach leaves, peas and pepper and cook for a further 2–3 minutes.

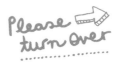

Please
turn over

To assemble the dumplings, remove the dough from the refrigerator. Take a dough circle in your hand, wet the edges and spoon a heaped teaspoon of the meat mixture into the centre. Fold the pastry in half and squeeze the sides together to seal. You can also pleat if you want to make them look more traditional and pretty.

To cook, drizzle the pan with a little extra sesame oil and heat over a medium heat. Add all of the dumplings to the pan and cook without turning for about 3 minutes. The bottom of the dumpling touching the pan should be browned.

Add the boiling water to the pan and cover with a lid to seal. The dumplings need to steam in the water for about 3 minutes. The dough should become translucent when cooked.

Serve with Toddler-Friendly Asian Dip (see page 204).

Potato Farls

It is worth peeling and cooking a few extra potatoes on a Sunday if it means you'll have leftovers to make potato farls. It's a simple dish that goes so well with Healthy Baked Beans (see page 78) and is perfect for little hands.

Makes 8 farls

450g cooked mashed potato

80g plain flour, plus extra for rolling

1 tablespoon melted butter

1 clove garlic, crushed

sprig of fresh rosemary, leaves picked and finely chopped

unsalted butter, to serve

Place the potato, flour and melted butter in a bowl and add the garlic and rosemary. Mix until it's fully combined and has become a smooth dough.

Turn out onto a well-floured surface and shape the dough into a circle about 2cm thick then cut into 8 equal parts.

Fry both sides of each part on a dry pan until golden brown.

Spread a little butter on one side to serve.

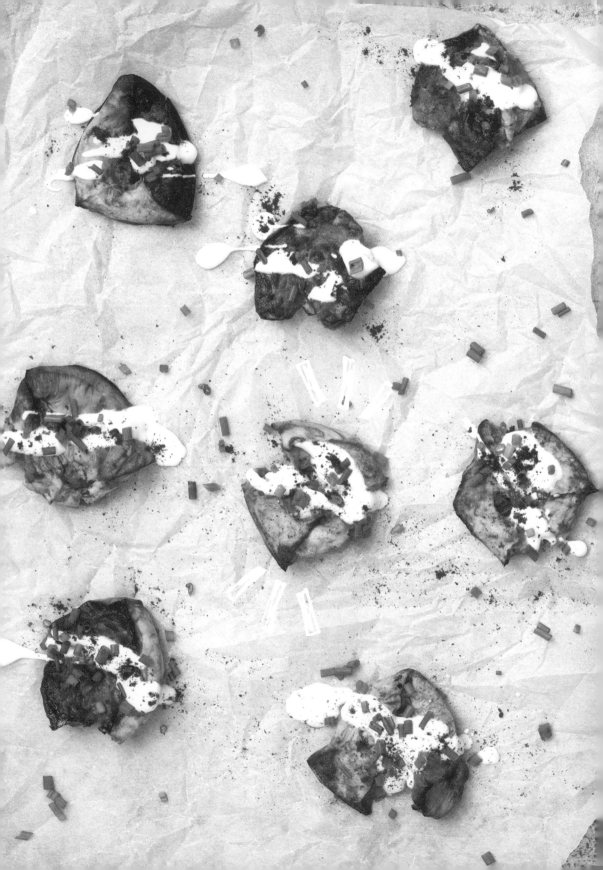

Roasted Smashed
Sweet Potatoes

This is our go-to recipe for a quick and tasty lunch that can be enjoyed by the entire family. You can also serve it with some beef or chicken and green vegetables to make a perfect dinner. It is cheap to make and so easy.

Serves 2 adults and 1 child

1 large sweet potato, peeled and cut into chunks

2 tablespoons olive oil

4 cloves garlic

4 tablespoons Greek yogurt

½ lemon, zest and juice

1 teaspoon smoked paprika

10 chives, finely chopped

Preheat oven to 160°C/325°F/gas 3.

Place the sweet potato on a baking tray, then drizzle with the olive oil and bake for 30 minutes or until soft. After around 15 minutes, add the whole cloves of garlic to the tray and cook with the potato. When cooked, remove from the oven and leave aside.

Meanwhile, add the yogurt and lemon to a bowl. Crush the soft roasted garlic into the bowl and stir really well.

Lightly squash each of the potato pieces and drizzle them with the yogurt sauce. Sprinkle a little paprika and a few chives on top of each one.

Serve warm.

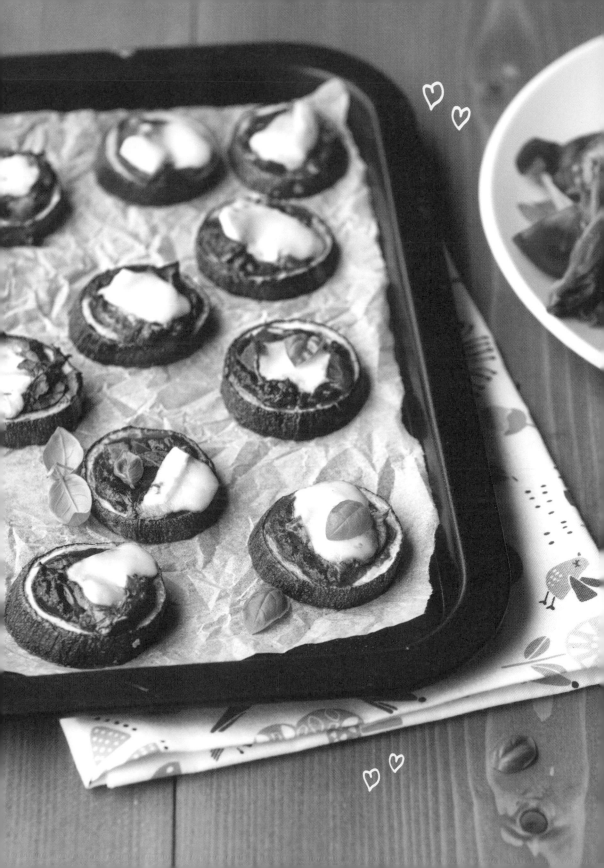

Courgette Pizzas

One of the most delicious ways you will ever taste courgette and one of the best ways to get your little ones eating them – especially if they don't like them to begin with. Each bite is a little piece of heaven and they are full of healthy goodness and wonderful flavours.

Makes 12 slices

1 medium courgette, cut into 12 thick slices

1 tablespoon tomato purée

1 small clove garlic, crushed

½ tablespoon olive oil

½ tablespoon water

8 basil leaves, finely chopped

2 cherry tomatoes, finely chopped

50g mozzarella, chopped into small pieces

Preheat oven to 180°C/350°F/gas 4.

Press down the centre of each courgette slice, so that it has a little dip for the filling. Place on a lightly oiled baking tray and bake for 10 minutes. Then remove and leave aside.

While the courgettes are cooking add the tomato purée, garlic, oil, water and basil to a bowl and stir well until it forms a thick sauce.

Spoon a little of the sauce onto each courgette slice and place a few pieces of tomato and one piece of mozarella on top.

Bake for 10 minutes, just enough time to allow the cheese to melt. The courgette shouldn't be too soft, just firm enough for your little one to hold but soft enough to squash if pressed.

Serve warm.

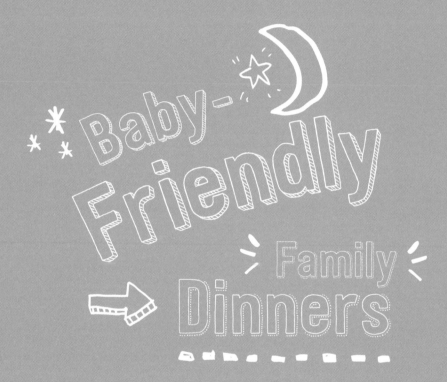

Baby-Friendly Family Dinners

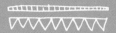

Eating dinner

as a family is one of the best ways to encourage
healthy eating habits that will last a lifetime.
Besides enjoying all the laughing and talking
about your day, your little one will join
in with the fun and want what you are eating.
All of the recipes in this section are
baby-friendly family meals,
so you can cook one meal that everyone can
enjoy.

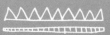

Avocado Pasta

This is a wonderfully simple dish that can be made in a jiffy on those days you want something healthy but don't want to spend long in the kitchen. The sauce is creamy, light and so nutritious. It's a great way to get some healthy fats in your little ones.

Serves 2 adults and 2 children

120g macaroni pasta

4 tablespoons olive oil

1 medium white onion, finely diced

2 cloves garlic, crushed

2 ripe avocados, halved and stones removed

½ lemon, juice only

15g fresh basil leaves, finely chopped

black pepper, to season

80g frozen peas

Cook the pasta as per the instructions on the pack. When soft, remove from the heat, drain and run some cold water over it to prevent it sticking together. Leave it aside while you make the sauce.

Heat the olive oil in a saucepan over a medium heat and gently fry the onion until soft. Add the garlic and cook for a further 2–3 minutes.

Add the onion mixture and avocados to a blender with the lemon juice and half of the basil leaves and blend until smooth and creamy. Add a little pepper to lightly season. Then pour the sauce back into the saucepan, add the pasta and frozen peas and stir well. Bring to a simmer, then pour into bowls and decorate with the remaining basil leaves.

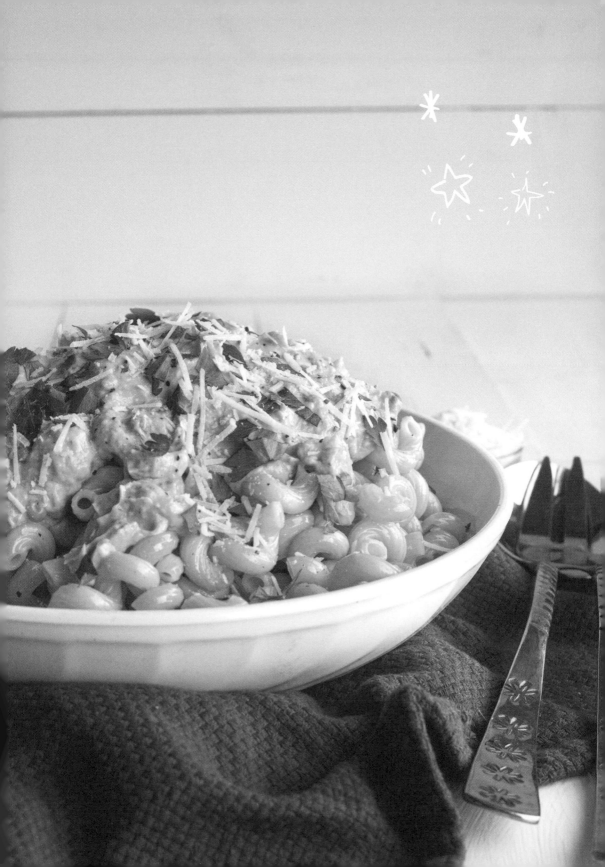

Butternut Squash
Pasta

This is one of the most popular recipes on my blog. When you make it, you will be surprised to see how deliciously creamy a sauce can be without using cream or butter – kids love it!

Serves 2 adults and 2 children

1 small butternut squash, peeled, deseeded and cut into chunks

2 tablespoons olive oil, plus extra for frying

1 medium onion, finely chopped

2 cloves garlic, crushed

pinch black pepper

125ml vegetable stock or water

1 tablespoon natural yogurt

250g penne or fusilli pasta

Preheat oven to 180°C/350°F/gas 4.

Place the chopped butternut squash on a baking sheet, drizzle with the olive oil and roast for about 40 minutes (or until soft).

Heat a drizzle of olive oil in a frying pan and gently fry the onion until it starts to turn sweet and sticky. This takes about 10 minutes but it's so worth it.

Add the garlic to the pan and cook for a further 3 or so minutes, stirring well to make sure it doesn't burn. Add the roasted butternut squash and all the remaining ingredients (except for the pasta) to the pan, reduce the heat and simmer for 10 minutes.

While the sauce is cooking, bring a pot of water to the boil and cook your pasta as per the package instructions. When the pasta is cooked, drain and leave to the side.

Add all of the sauce ingredients to a blender and blend until smooth and creamy, then pour over your pasta, stirring well to coat each and every piece.

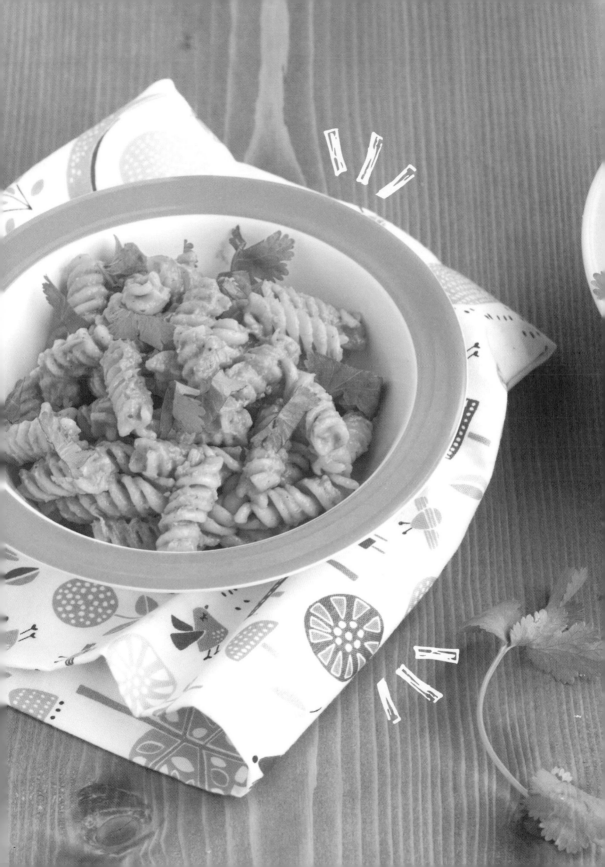

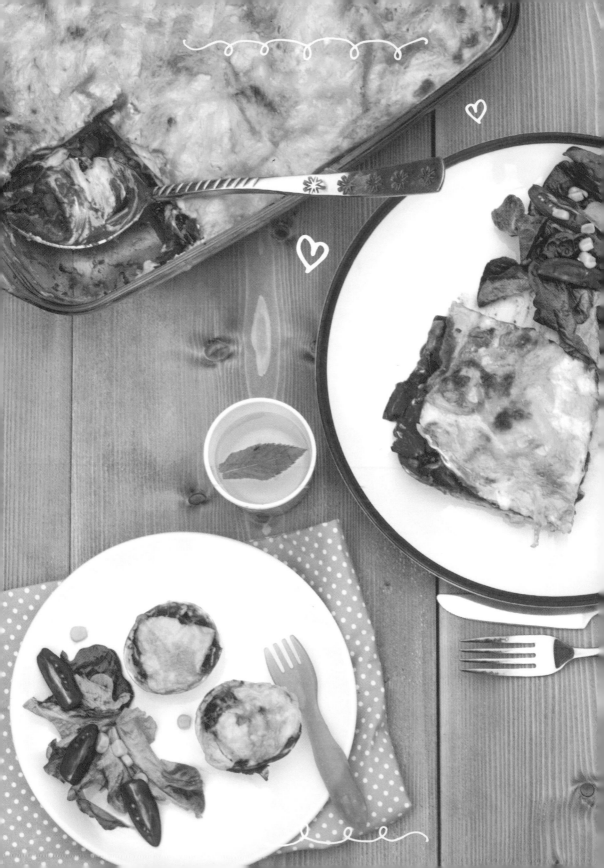

Roasted Vegetable
Mini-Lasagnes

We try to eat vegetarian at least half the week, and I try to be creative in how I get the kiddies to eat their veggies. There has never been any fuss about this dish, though – everything is soft and delicious and, with the mini-lasagnes for the little one, it is an ideal baby-friendly family meal.

Makes 1 family-sized and 12 baby lasagnes

1 aubergine, sliced thinly lengthways

2 courgettes, sliced thinly lengthways

3 red peppers, thinly sliced

1 bulb garlic

2 tablespoons olive oil, plus extra for roasting

1 large white onion, finely chopped

400g tinned tomatoes

3 tablespoons unsalted tomato purée

15 basil leaves, finely chopped

2 teaspoons apple cider vinegar

¼ teaspoon English mustard

50g unsalted butter

2 tablespoons flour

260ml milk

150g cheddar cheese, grated, plus extra for sprinkling

500g fresh lasagne sheets

Preheat oven to 200°C/400°F/gas 6.

Place the aubergine, courgette and pepper slices on two baking trays lined with parchment paper and drizzle with a little olive oil. Break up the bulb of garlic – but don't remove the cloves from their skins – and add to the vegetables. Roast for 20 minutes until everything is soft and then remove from the oven. For the baby portions, take about a quarter of the vegetables and a few cloves of garlic. Remove the skins from the garlic and finely chop it and the vegetables.

Heat 2 tablespoons of olive oil in a saucepan and fry the onion on a medium heat for about 8 minutes, stirring regularly. Add the tin of tomatoes, tomato purée, basil, apple cider vinegar and mustard and stir well. Simmer over a low heat for about 10 minutes until the sauce becomes a rich red. Then remove from the heat and leave aside until you are ready to assemble the lasagnes.

To make the cheese sauce, melt the butter in a small saucepan over a medium to low heat. Slowly add the flour and stir continuously until a paste forms. Cook this over a low heat for about 2 minutes.

Gradually pour in the milk, whisking each addition into the sauce before adding more. Take your time to prevent the sauce from becoming lumpy. If your sauce is too thick, add a little more milk until you get the right consistency. Add the cheese and stir until it fully melts.

Please turn over

Courgette Noodles
with Pesto

Courgettes are such a versatile vegetable, and when served as courgette spaghetti, they are transformed into a delicious vegetable noodle that kids love. For a really tasty family meal, I serve these with pesto, a few roasted cherry tomatoes and some thin slices of fresh buffalo mozzarella.

Serves 2 adults and 2 children

4 courgettes

1 tablespoon olive oil

½ lemon, juice only

pepper, to season

80ml Spinach and Kale Pesto (see page 200)

18 cherry tomatoes, roasted

125g buffalo mozzarella, sliced

Make the veggie noodles by using a julienne peeler or spiraliser. Then place into a large bowl and drizzle over the olive oil, lemon juice and pepper. Use your hands to make sure that the noodles are completely coated.

Heat a frying pan over a medium heat, add the noodles and stir-fry for about 3 minutes. They should be soft and heated the whole way through but not overcooked.

Add the pesto to the pan, give it a good stir and pour into a large serving bowl. Top with the cherry tomatoes and mozzarella.

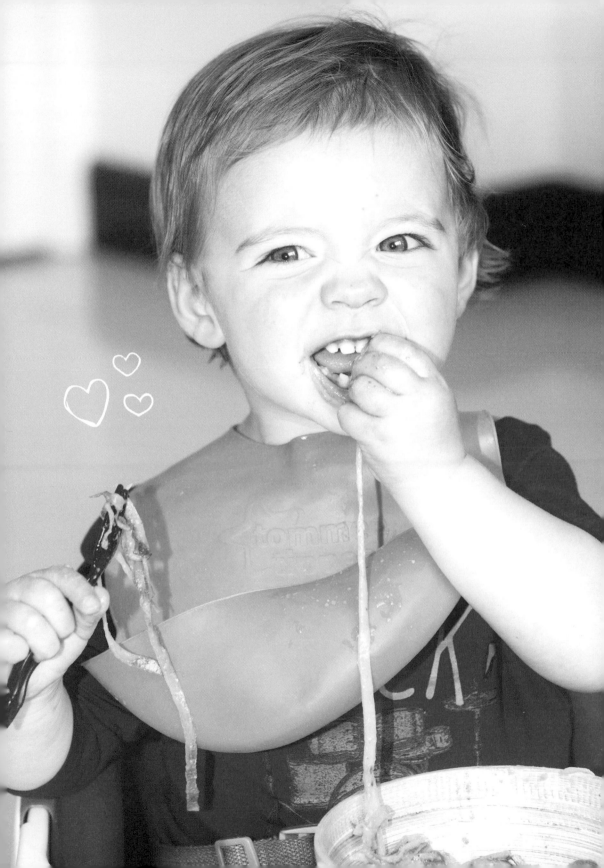

Mac 'n' Cheesey
Baby Muffins

Mac and cheese is the ultimate comfort food – a creamy white, cheesy sauce clinging to softly cooked macaroni and topped with crispy breadcrumbs. This recipe is my take on the traditional American dish and they look so cute when cooked in a mini-muffin tin. I make a big batch and freeze as they are handy for busy evenings.

Makes 24 mini-muffins

260g macaroni pasta

50g unsalted butter

2 tablespoons flour

250ml milk

125g cheddar cheese, grated

½ teaspoon ground nutmeg

black pepper, to season

1 slice wholemeal bread, blitzed into crumbs

Preheat oven to 200°C/400°F/gas 6.

Cook the pasta according to the instructions on the pack. When soft, drain and leave aside while you make the sauce.

Melt the butter in a saucepan over a low heat, then whisk in the flour and stir well until it forms a roux (or paste). Keep stirring for a further 2 minutes to allow the flour to cook in the butter and then, very slowly, add the milk a little at a time, making sure to stir vigorously as you do to prevent lumps. Keep going until all the milk has been incorporated, then remove the sauce from the heat and stir in the cheese, nutmeg and pepper. Stir well until the cheese has fully melted.

Add the cooked pasta to the sauce and mix well, then spoon the mixture into a well-oiled mini-muffin tin for smaller babies or a regular muffin tin for older toddlers.

Sprinkle the top of each muffin with breadcrumbs and bake at 200°C for 25 minutes.

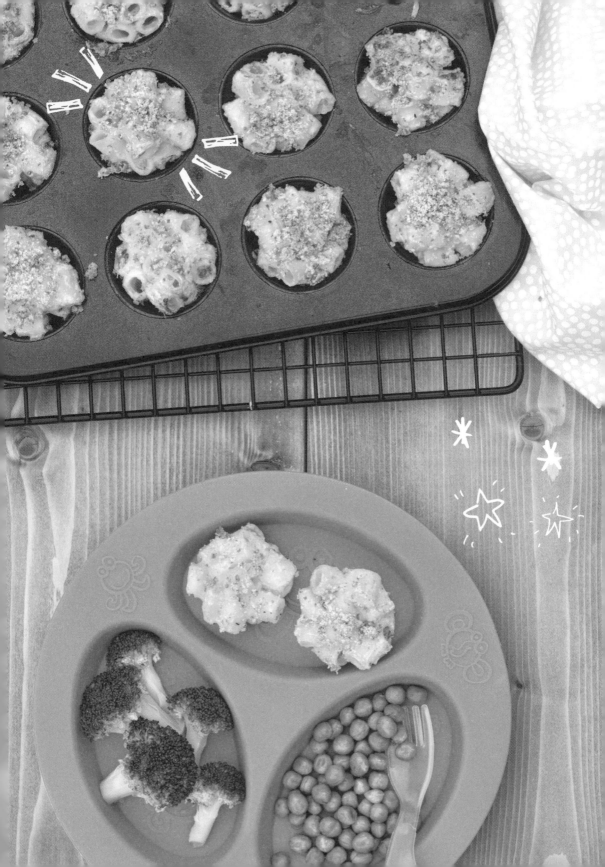

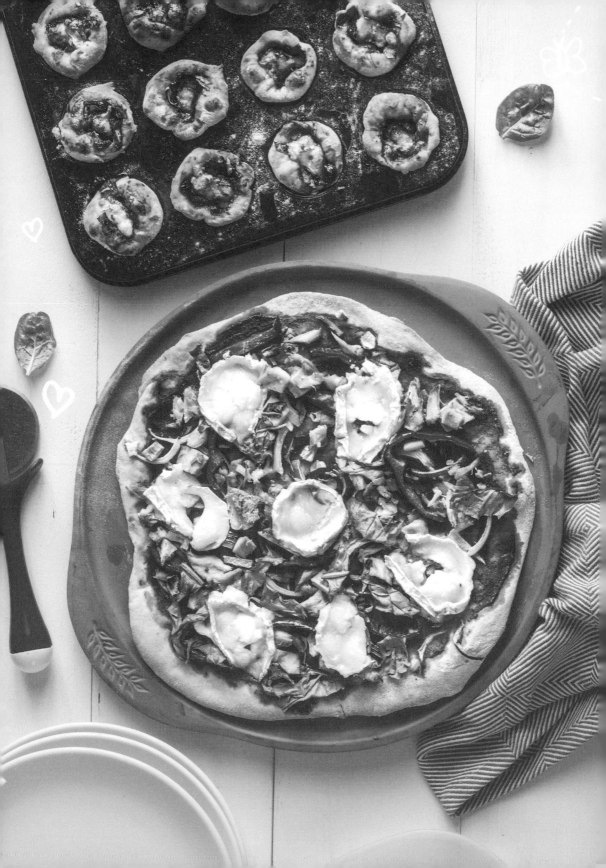

Gourmet Family
Pizza

On any given day, if I was to ask my children what their dream dinner would be, they would always answer pizza! Making homemade pizzas is a fun thing to do with kids, from rolling out the dough to adorning their own pizza with the veggies they have picked themselves. They are ideal to have in the freezer and defrost in less than an hour.

Makes 24 baby and 3 adult pizzas

2 tsp (10g): 6g free sugar
(24 servings) 0.25g each

For the pizza dough

250ml warm water

3 tablespoons olive oil

7g fast-acting dried yeast

2 teaspoons maple syrup

320g strong white flour

For the quick pizza sauce

150g unsalted tomato purée

1 clove garlic, crushed

4 tablespoons water

1 teaspoon dried oregano

For the pizza toppings

1 large onion, sliced

2 handfuls baby leaf spinach, finely chopped (for baby pizzas)

10 button mushrooms, finely chopped

2 red bell peppers (for adult pizzas)

2 packs buffalo mozzarella

2 cooked chicken breasts roughly chopped

To make the dough, add the warm water and olive oil to a jug, then stir in the yeast and maple syrup and whisk until fully combined. Leave aside for about 10 minutes until the yeast activates. It should be frothy on top.

Sieve the flour into a large bowl and make a well in the middle of it. You can also use a food mixer with a dough hook (I like the workout so I do it the harder way).

Slowly add your water and yeast mix and stir it in using your hands, if not using a machine, until the flour and water are fully combined and you are left with a dough.

Turn it out onto a well-floured counter top, cover your hands with flour and knead until soft and springy. This takes a good 10 minutes but it is quite therapeutic and great fun to do with kids.

When you've finished kneading, you need to let it prove. Place the dough in a floured bowl covered with a towel or cling film in a warm place for an hour. It should double in size. (While your dough is proving you can make your sauce and get the fillings ready.)

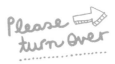

Please
turn over

When proved, turn the dough back out onto a floured surface and knead it again, but only for a few moments – you just want to remove the air from it. Cut the dough into 4 parts – 3 for adult pizzas and 1 for the 24 baby-bite pizzas.

To make the sauce, place all of the ingredients into a bowl and whisk together.

When you're ready to make the baby pizzas, preheat the oven to 200°C/400°F/gas 6.

Take a cherry-tomato-sized piece of dough and roll it out flat. Place in a mini-muffin tin, making sure the sides come right up. Add a teaspoon of sauce. (I like to add the sauce as I go along as it helps stop the dough from springing back up.) Do this for all 24 little pizzas.

Add a little spinach and chopped mushroom into each one and then top with a tiny piece of mozzarella.

Bake for about 12–15 minutes or until the dough is cooked underneath.

For the adult pizzas, preheat the oven to its hottest setting.

Roll each piece of dough out as flat as you can. If you can do this without a rolling pin, I'm super impressed!

Place each one on a baking tray or pizza stone, add a couple of tablespoons of sauce, sprinkle with toppings and place some mozzarella on top.

Bake for 10–12 minutes or until cooked underneath and no longer doughy.

Meatloaf Muffins

When I lived in San Francisco, this was one of my favourite things to cook for my daughter. It is one of the simplest dishes and is really just a lot of goodness mixed together into a delicious mouthful. Serve with some lovely creamy mashed spuds for the ultimate comfort food.

Makes 24 mini-muffins plus 1 loaf

2 tablespoons rapeseed oil

1 medium white onion, finely chopped

2 cloves garlic, crushed

2 red bell peppers, finely diced

4 tablespoons unsalted tomato purée

80ml water

400g minced beef

2 eggs

80g breadcrumbs

sprig of fresh thyme, leaves picked and finely chopped

1 teaspoon Dijon mustard

2 tablespoons parsley, finely chopped, plus extra to serve

125ml Baby Ketchup (see page 203)

Preheat oven to 180°C/350°F/gas 4.

Heat the oil in a saucepan and gently cook the onion for 3–4 minutes until translucent. Add the garlic, stir well and cook for another 2 minutes.

Add the peppers, tomato purée and water and mix well. Cook until the peppers are soft – this should only take 5 minutes or so because the pieces are so small. Take the pan off the heat and pour mixture into a large bowl.

Add the beef, eggs, breadcrumbs, thyme, mustard and parsley to the bowl and mix really well.

Oil a mini-muffin tin. Then take about a tablespoon of the mixture in the palm of your hand. Roll into a little ball and press into the mini-muffin tin. Do this until each of the 24 compartments is full, and then lightly spread a half-teaspoon of ketchup over the top of each muffin.

Place the remaining meat mixture into a 1lb loaf tin lined with parchment paper and spread the rest of the ketchup on top.

Place the muffins and the meatloaf tin in the oven.

Bake the muffins for 40 minutes. Bake the larger loaf for 1 hour.

Serve with a little fresh parsley sprinkled over and fluffy mashed potatoes.

Potato Gnocchi with Roasted Red Pepper Pesto

When you taste these homemade gnocchi and see how easy they are to make, I promise you, you will never buy the packaged kind again. These pillowy potato bites take less than 15 minutes to make and are delicious served with a little red pepper pesto. You will feel like you're in your favourite Italian restaurant with your little one by your side after the very first bite.

Serves 2 adults and 2 children

For the gnocchi

400g cold mashed potato

150g plain flour

1 medium-sized egg

pinch of pepper

2 tablespoons rapeseed oil (optional)

For the pesto

2 red bell peppers, roasted

60ml olive oil

4 cloves garlic, roasted

80g pumpkin seeds

20g hard goat's cheese, grated

1 tablespoon fresh oregano, chopped

black pepper, to season

To make the gnocchi, add the potato, flour, egg and pepper to a bowl and mix until fully combined. If the dough is too sticky you can add a little extra flour. Turn out onto a well-floured surface and divide into 6 pieces.

Roll each piece into a long log shape, roughly 2cm thick, and then cut into 2.5cm pieces. Take each little gnocchi and, using the back of a fork, press the flat part of the prongs onto the dough to add little dents. This will help the sauce to cling when cooked.

Half fill a saucepan with water and bring to the boil. Add the gnocchi in batches and cook each batch for about 3 minutes. They are cooked when they rise to the surface. Using a slotted spoon, remove from the water. You can serve them like this but, to make them easier for little hands, I fry them for a few minutes to make them less slippy. Simply heat the oil over a medium heat and add in batches. Cook on both sides until golden.

To make the pesto, place all of the ingredients in a blender and whizz until smooth and silky. Heat gently in a saucepan and pour over gnocchi to serve.

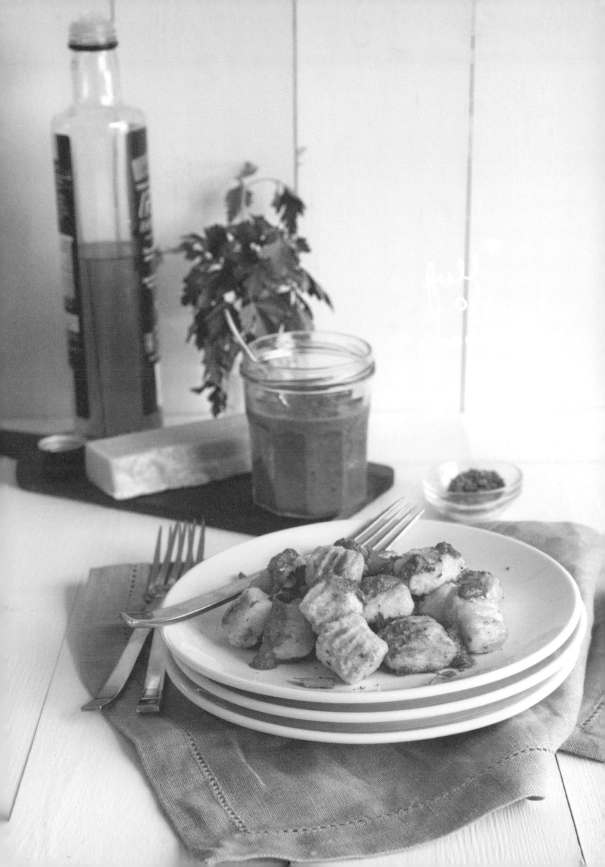

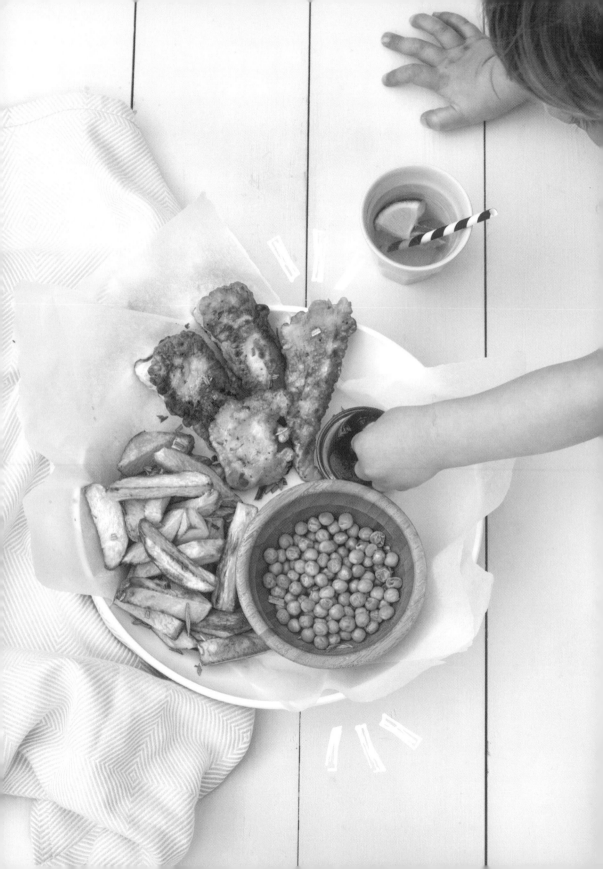

Fish 'n' Chips

This is one sure way I know of getting my kids to eat fish. Yes, it is fried, but in healthy oil and the chips are baked so it is a healthier version of traditional fish and chips. Hake is delicious and when bought fresh over the counter you can be sure of a flaky and meaty fish very similar to cod. While you're at the fish counter, ask them to take the skin off as it is much easier than trying to do it at home.

Serves 2 adults and 2 children

6 medium-sized potatoes (preferably Maris Piper), washed

4 tablespoons rapeseed oil, plus extra for frying fish

500g hake fillet or other white fish, bones removed carefully

100g flour, plus 4 tablespoons extra for coating fish

black pepper, to season

180ml milk

60ml rapeseed oil

sprig fresh rosemary, leaves picked and finely chopped

Preheat oven to 160°C/325°F/gas 3.

Cut the potatoes into large wedges. Place them in a bowl, then add the rapeseed oil and, using your hands, rub it all over the wedges until they are fully coated. Line a baking tray with parchment paper and place the wedges skin-side down in rows. Bake in the oven for roughly 30 minutes or until golden and cooked through.

Meanwhile, cut the hake into baby-sized portions.

Add the flour and pepper to a large bowl. Make a well in the centre and slowly whisk in the milk until it becomes a smooth batter.

In a separate large bowl, place the additional flour.

Heat the rapeseed oil in a frying pan over a high heat, then work quickly to batter the fish.

Dip each piece of fish into the flour, shake off any excess, then dip into the batter and place on the pan. I cook about 3 pieces at a time.

When the fish is browned on each side, remove and place on paper towels to remove any excess oil. Keep frying off the fish until it is all cooked.

When you are ready to serve, sprinkle the rosemary over the chips. Serve with a little wedge of lemon, Baby Ketchup (see page 203) and peas.

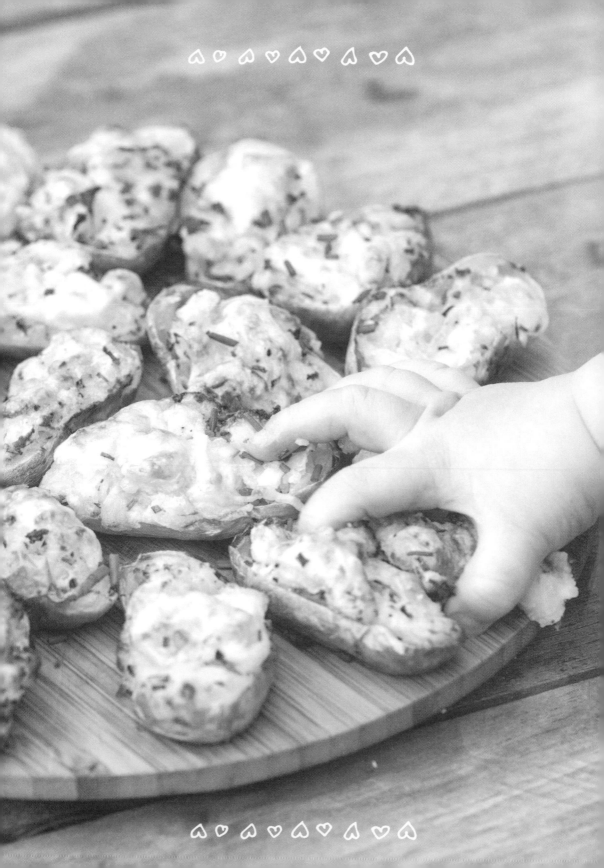

Cheese & Chive Stuffed
Baby Potatoes

Baby potatoes are ideal for small hands and make a perfect weaning food. They are soft, nutritious and filling for little tummies. For babies starting out, I give half a potato and for older babies two halves. Serve with some roast chicken or lamb for the perfect little meal.

Makes 24

12 baby potatoes

50ml milk

1 tablespoon unsalted butter

2 shallots, finely chopped

100g broccoli, steamed and finely chopped

100ml sour cream

12 chives, finely chopped

¼ teaspoon ground nutmeg

100g cheddar cheese, grated

Heat oven to 200°C/400°F/gas 6.

Prick the baby potatoes with a fork before placing on an oven tray and baking for approximately 40 minutes (or until soft).

Allow the cooked potatoes to cool fully. Then cut them in half long ways and scoop out the soft potato into a bowl, leaving the skins aside for later.

Add the milk and butter to the potato and mash until smooth.

Add the shallots, broccoli, sour cream, chives and nutmeg and stir until everything is full combined.

Spoon the filling into each of the reserved potato skins and lay on a baking tray.

Sprinkle each one with a little cheese and bake for 25–30 minutes until golden.

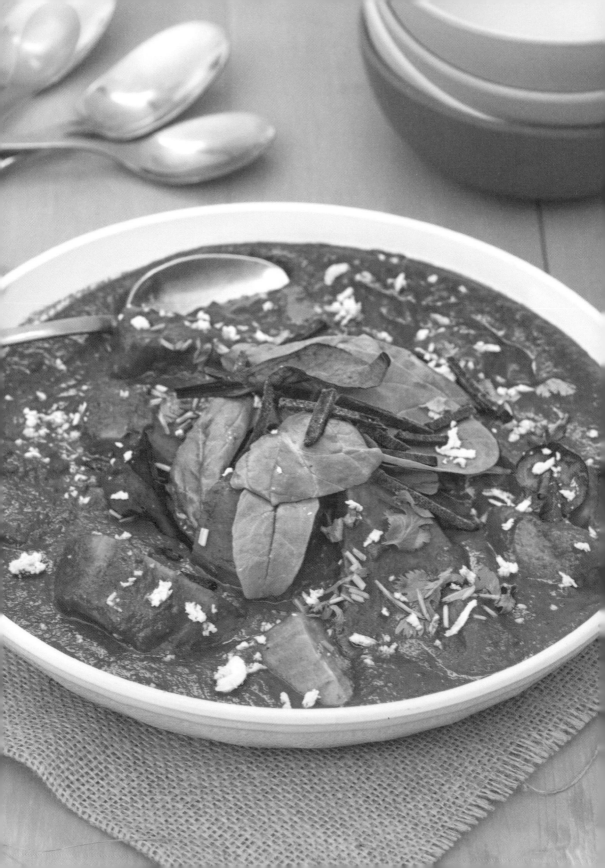

Sweet Potato Curry

This curry is deliciously creamy and packs a punch of spice and flavour. The sauce reduces down so that the sweet potato is not only soft but also easy for babies to pick up and feed themselves. It can get messy, so make sure you have a long-sleeved bib on your little one to save on the washing!

Serves 2 adults and 2 children

2 tablespoons olive or rapeseed oil

1 medium white onion, roughly chopped

4 cloves garlic, crushed

4 tablespoons unsalted tomato purée

400g tinned chopped tomatoes

400ml coconut milk

1 stick lemongrass, peeled and finely chopped

1 teaspoon ground paprika

1 teaspoon ground cumin

1 teaspoon ground coriander

1 teaspoon garam masala

½ teaspoon turmeric

2 large sweet potatoes, peeled and cut into chunks

bunch fresh coriander, finely chopped, to garnish

Heat the oil in a pan over a medium heat and fry the onion, stirring often, until it starts to caramelise. This should take about 8 minutes. Add the garlic and fry for 2 minutes until soft but not browning.

Add the tomato purée, chopped tomatoes, coconut milk, lemongrass and spices.

Using a stick blender, blend the sauce until smooth and creamy. Then add the sweet potatoes to the pan.

Turn the heat to low, cover the saucepan and leave to cook for about 20 minutes. Then remove the lid and cook for a further 20 minutes to allow the sauce to thicken.

Sprinkle with chopped coriander and some spinach and beetroot (optional). Serve with cooked brown rice or naan bread.

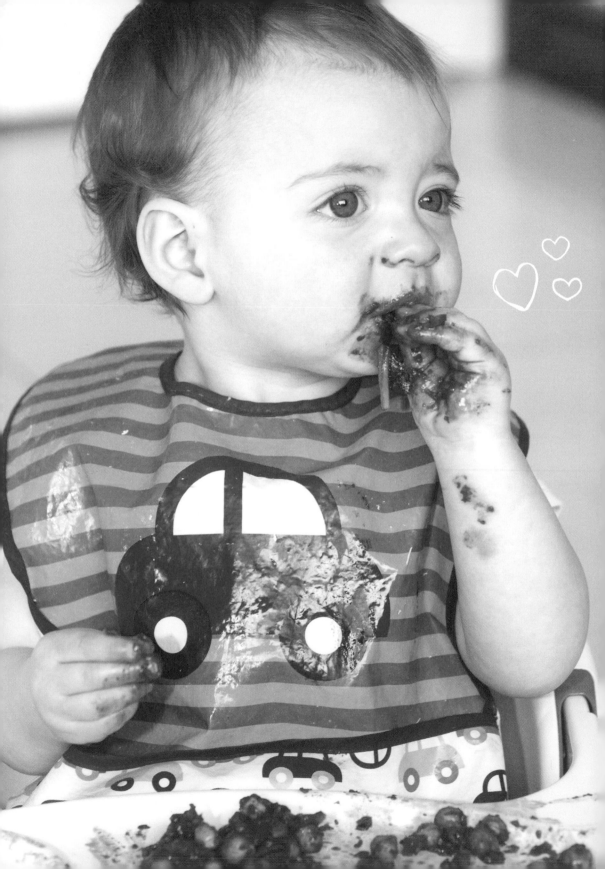

Moroccan Spiced
Chickpeas

A super-healthy mix of spices and chickpeas in a tomato sauce makes up our ultimate curry-in-a-hurry. Chickpeas are wonderful little powerhouses of nutrition, and if your family love curry, they will love this recipe.

Serves 2 adults and 2 children

2 tablespoons rapeseed oil

1 large white onion, finely chopped

2 cloves garlic, crushed

1 teaspoon ground cumin

1 teaspoon ground coriander

½ teaspoon turmeric

½ teaspoon ground ginger

½ teaspoon ground cinnamon

4 cardamon pods, deseeded and seeds crushed

4 tablespoons tomato purée

400g tinned tomatoes

800g tinned chickpeas

80ml water

4 large handfuls baby leaf spinach, chopped

black pepper, to season

Heat the oil in a saucepan over a medium heat. Gently fry the onion for 6 minutes, stirring often, until it turns lovely and golden. Add the garlic and fry for another couple of minutes.

Add the spices and tomato purée and stir well. Allow to cook for a few minutes until the spices become lovely and fragrant. Then add the tinned tomatoes, chickpeas and water and turn the heat down to a simmer. Leave the lid off the pot and allow the sauce to reduce until thickened. This only takes about 10 minutes. Remove from the heat and add the spinach leaves, along with a little pepper to season.

Serve with homemade tortillas (see page 143).

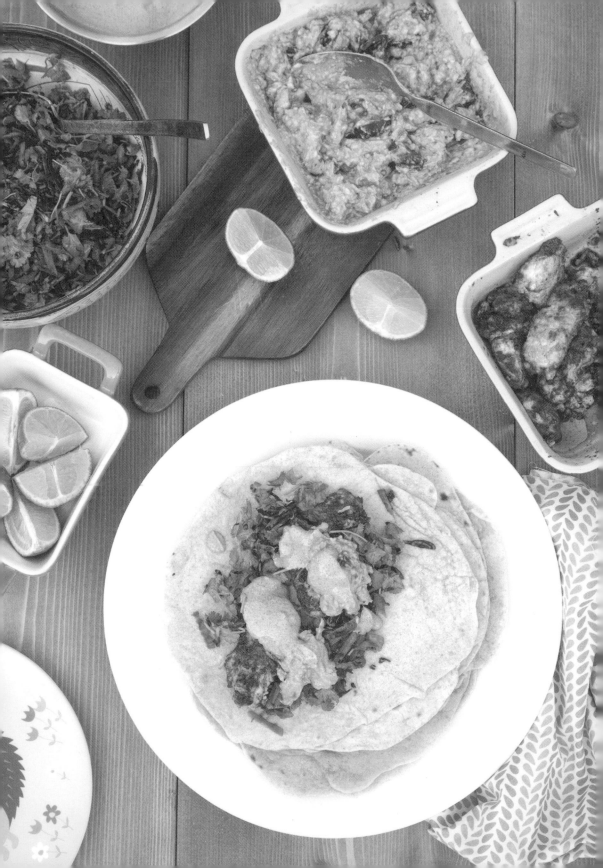

Fish Tacos
with Homemade Slaw & Flour Tortillas

My friend and amazing food photographer Ed Anderson made this dish for me recently when I visited their home in San Francisco. He never gave me his spice-mix recipe but I conjured up my own version and the kids just loved it! It's a great way to eat fish and looks so impressive when laid out on the table – yet it takes less than 30 minutes to prepare.

Serves 2 adults and 2 children

For the tortillas
280g plain flour

1 teaspoon baking powder

160ml cold water

3 tablespoons rapeseed oil

For the fish
400g hake, cut into bite-sized pieces and any bones removed

1 teaspoon paprika

1 teaspoon ground cumin

1 teaspoon ground coriander

black pepper, to season

1 lime, juice only

2 tablespoons rapeseed oil

For the slaw
100g red cabbage, grated

100g carrot, grated

4 tablespoons natural yogurt

1 lime, juice only

small bunch fresh coriander, finely chopped

To make the flour tortillas, mix the flour and baking powder in a large bowl. Make a well in the centre and pour in the water and oil. Using your hands, work into a dough. Then turn it out onto a floured surface and knead for just a few minutes. Divide the dough into 16 parts and roll out into circles.

Heat a dry pan over a medium heat. Place a tortilla in the pan and cook until you see bubbles forming. Then flip it over and cook the other side. It should take about a minute each side. Wrap in a dry, clean tea-towel and leave aside. Repeat, adding each cooked tortilla to the tea-towel, until all of the tortillas are done.

Next, place the fish in a bowl, along with the spices and lime juice. Use your hands to make sure each piece is fully coated in the spice mixture.

Heat the rapeseed oil in a pan over a medium heat and then fry the fish until browned on both sides and cooked through. It should only take about 10 minutes.

Meanwhile, place the cabbage and carrot in a large bowl along with the yogurt and lime. Mix and sprinkle the fresh coriander over.

Divide the fish between the warm tortillas, spoon over a little slaw and serve with guacamole (see page 201) and Cajun Sauce (see page 204)

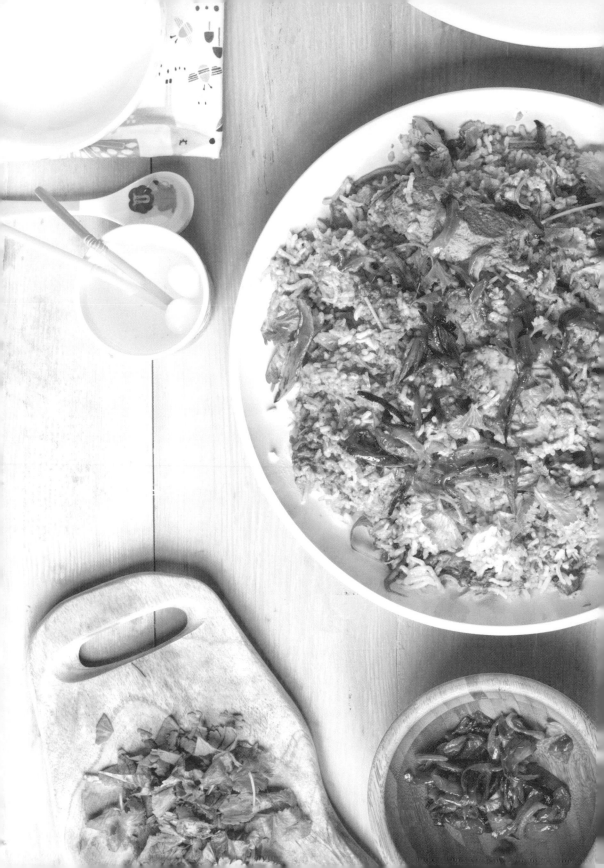

Tandoori Chicken Biryani

Biryani is a lovely dish for little ones, as the chicken is so tender it breaks up easily and the rice is easy for them to shovel into their little mouths. This dish is a great way to introduce new flavours like ginger and other spices too. Marinate the chicken the night before for best results.

Serves 2 adults and 2 children

For the chicken marinade

5 free-range chicken fillets, cut into long strips

3 medium white onions

6 cloves garlic

20g ginger root, peeled

200ml natural yogurt

1 teaspoon ground cumin

1 teaspoon ground coriander

1 teaspoon smoked paprika

1 teaspoon turmeric

2 teaspoons garam masala

3 tablespoons tomato purée

6 cardamon pods, seeds only

bunch of fresh coriander stalks (put leaves aside for garnish)

For the rice

200g basmati rice

480ml water

½ teaspoon ground cloves

4 cardamon pods, seeds only

¼ teaspoon ground cinnamon

For the fried onions

60ml rapeseed oil

2 large white onions, chopped

4 tablespoons ghee or rapeseed oil

4 tablespoons water

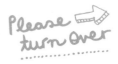
Please turn over

Place the chicken strips in a bowl.

Add the rest of the ingredients for the marinade to a blender and blend into a smooth, creamy sauce.

Pour the sauce over the chicken and, using your hands, make sure that every piece of the chicken is completely coated. Cover the bowl with cling film and leave to marinate in the fridge for at least 4 hours but preferably overnight.

For perfectly fluffy rice, place the rice in a bowl, cover with water and leave overnight as well.

When you are ready to cook, preheat the oven to 160°C/325°F/gas 3.

Pour the chicken onto a tray lined with parchment paper, making sure that there is a little space between each piece. Bake for 30 minutes until the chicken is fully cooked through.

Meanwhile, pour the rice into a sieve and rinse under the tap until the water runs clear. Put the rice into a saucepan with the 480ml water, cloves, cardamom seeds and cinnamon and then bring the water to the boil. Give it a good stir, place a lid on the saucepan and turn the heat to its lowest setting. Leave for 10 minutes before removing the lid.

While the rice is cooking, heat the rapeseed oil in a frying pan and fry the onions until golden and sticky, making sure to stir often. This will take about 10 minutes – just be careful not to burn them. When they are cooked, place them on kitchen paper to remove any extra oil.

To make the biryani, start by adding the ghee or rapeseed oil to a large pot along with the water. Heat gently so that the ghee melts, and then add a third of the chicken mixture followed by a third of the rice on top and then sprinkle with a third of the fried onions. Repeat until all of the chicken, rice and onion are used up. You should be left with some sauce on the baking tray from the chicken. I add a little boiling water to this to loosen it up and then pour it over the rice.

Place the pot over a medium heat until you see steam coming up through the rice. Then place a lid on it and simmer for about 30 minutes.

To serve, empty into a large bowl and sprinkle with the fresh coriander leaves.

Thai Chicken
Curry Noodles

Another speedy dish! It takes all of 5 minutes to prepare the curry paste, throw in the coconut milk, meat and other ingredients and, hey presto, a delicious Thai-inspired curry the entire family will love. I like to roast a few chillies in some foil to add to my own plate, and that's really it – everyone's happy, job done!

Serves 2 adults and 2 children

1 tbsp (20g): 12.1g free sugar
(4 servings) 3g each

For the curry paste

2 cloves garlic, peeled

2 shallots, peeled

10g ginger root, peeled

1 teaspoon ground coriander

1 teaspoon ground cumin

½ teaspoon ground cinnamon

1 teaspoon turmeric

1 teaspoon fish sauce

2 tablespoons water

3 tablespoons rapeseed oil

For the curry

1 tin coconut milk

4 chicken breasts, cut into finger-sized strips

6 kaffir lime leaves (optional)

1 lime, juice only

1 tablespoon maple syrup

2 sticks lemongrass, peeled and finely chopped

1 pack soba noodles

Add all of the ingredients for the paste to a blender and blend until smooth.

Add the curry paste to a saucepan and cook for about 5 minutes, stirring all the time. It should turn lovely and fragrant.

Add the coconut milk and bring to a simmer. Then add the chicken and kaffir lime leaves, if using.

Leave the lid off the pot and turn the heat to low. Leave to simmer for about 20 minutes. The chicken should cook really slowly to ensure it is not chewy and will be tender for little babies.

Add the lime juice, maple syrup and lemongrass, and cook on low for another 20 minutes.

Cook the soba noodles according to the pack's instructions and serve the curry over the noodles.

Chicken Tikka with Sweet Potato Fries & Raita

This recipe is easy to make and so yummy that the kids devour it each and every time. If you can, marinate the chicken overnight, as the acid in the yogurt breaks down the chicken, making it much more tender.

Serves 2 adults and 2 children

For the chicken tikka

4 chicken breasts, cut into finger-sized strips

4 cloves garlic

7g ginger root

1 teaspoon turmeric

2 teaspoons ground coriander

2 teaspoons ground cumin

2 teaspoons paprika

1 teaspoon garam masala

½ teaspoon chilli powder (optional)

250ml natural yogurt

1 lemon, zest and juice

pinch black pepper

For the sweet potato fries

2 sweet potatoes, peeled and cut into spears

3 tablespoons olive oil

For the raita

240ml natural yogurt

4 cloves garlic, roasted and crushed

1 bunch fresh mint leaves (about 10g), finely chopped

pinch black pepper

½ teaspoon paprika

Place the chicken in a medium-sized bowl. Add the rest of the tikka ingredients to a blender and pulse until creamy and smooth. Pour over the chicken and, using a spatula or your hands, give everything a good mix to ensure the chicken is completely coated. Cover and leave in the fridge for at least 4 hours but preferably overnight.

When you're ready to cook, preheat the oven to 180°C/350°F/gas 4.

Place the sweet potatoes in a bowl, drizzle over the olive oil and, using your hands, give it a good mix to ensure the potatoes are fully coated. Place them onto a baking tray lined with parchment paper.

Remove the chicken from the fridge, turn it out onto another baking tray lined with parchment paper and bake both the sweet potato and chicken for 30 minutes. Halfway through, turn the pieces of chicken over.

While the chicken and potatoes are cooking, make the raita. Place the yogurt in a bowl and add the garlic and mint leaves. Add a little sprinkle of black pepper to taste and the paprika and give it a good stir.

Serve the chicken with the fries and the sauce drizzled over.

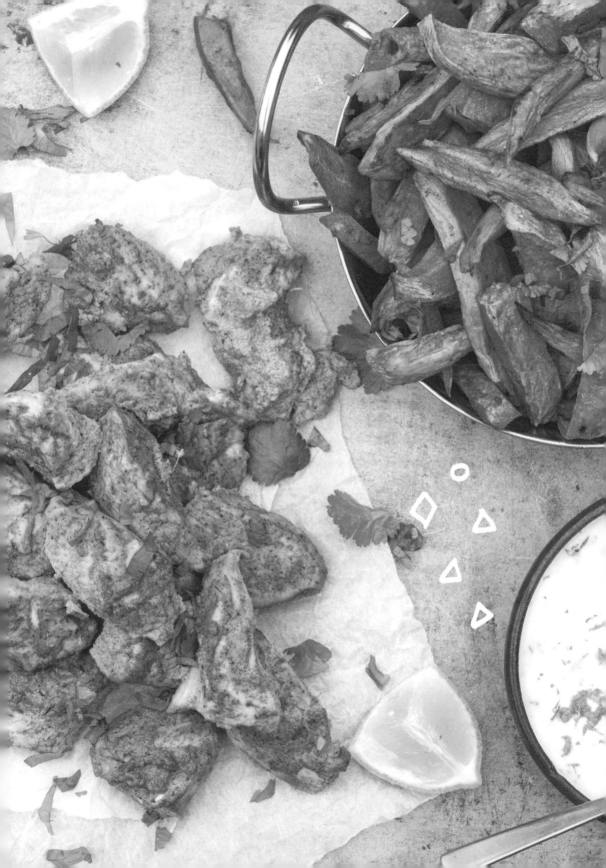

Chicken Korma Pies

While the grownups and big kids are munching away on a delicious, healthy chicken korma, your little one can get in on the action with super-cute korma pies. They are made using a shortcrust pastry filled with the exact same dish everyone else is having – it's just that bit less messy for little hands.

Serves 2 adults and 2 children, plus 24 mini-pies

For the chicken korma

2 tablespoons rapeseed oil

1 medium white onion, roughly chopped

2 cloves garlic, crushed

15g ginger root, finely chopped

400ml tinned coconut milk

80g sugar-free desiccated coconut

4 tablespoons ground almonds

4 tablespoons unsalted tomato purée

1 teaspoon ground cumin

1 teaspoon ground coriander

½ teaspoon turmeric

4 chicken breasts, cut into thin strips

6 cardamon pods, seeds only

5cm stick cinnamon

For the pastry

300g plain flour

150g butter

4 tablespoons water

1 egg, beaten

Heat the rapeseed oil in a saucepan over a medium heat and gently fry the onion for 3–4 minutes until it starts to turn translucent. Add the garlic and ginger and fry for 2 more minutes. Add the coconut milk, desiccated coconut, almonds, tomato purée and ground spices to the saucepan and give it a good stir. Once it starts to bubble, remove from the heat and, using a stick blender, blend until creamy and smooth.

Add the chicken to the sauce, along with the cardamon seeds and cinnamon. Turn the heat to low and leave the lid off to allow the chicken to gently cook and the sauce to thicken.

Meanwhile, preheat oven to 200°C/400°F/gas 6 and get started on the pastry.

Sieve the flour into a bowl and, using your fingers, work the butter in until the mixture starts to resemble fine breadcrumbs. Add the water a tablespoon at a time until the pastry comes together.

Place the pastry onto a lightly floured surface and roll until about half a centimetre thick. Cut out 24 circles to fit into a mini-muffin tin and 24 smaller lids to seal the little pies.

Lightly butter a mini-muffin tin and line each cup with a pastry case. When the chicken korma is cooked fully, fill each pastry case to the top with a little chicken and some sauce, then seal with the pie lid. Press down gently so that the pies are sealed. Beat the egg and lightly brush the pastry with it before baking for 25 minutes.

Serve the main dish with basmati rice or naan bread, while your little one munches away on their pie.

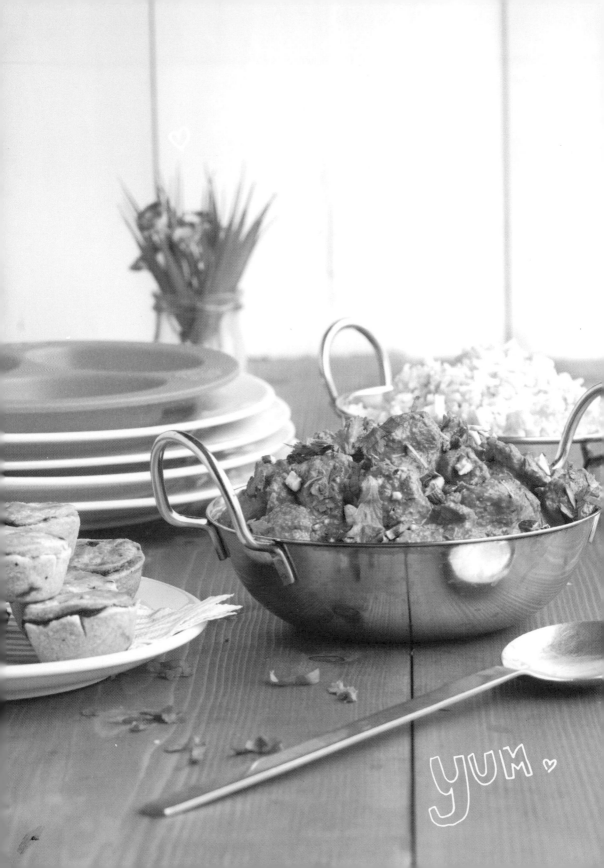

yum ♥

Pearl Barley with
Soft Roast Veggies & Orange Beef

This recipe is a delicious way to serve pearl barley – soft roasted vegetables with orange-glazed beef, all tossed with this deliciously soft and nutritious grain.

Serves 2 adults and 2 children

2 tbsp (40g): 24.2g free sugar
(4 servings) 6g each

For the roast vegetables

rapeseed oil, for drizzling

2 red bell peppers, roughly chopped

2 courgettes, roughly chopped

4 medium-sized onions, roughly chopped

1 bulb garlic, broken into cloves (skins left on)

For the barley

2 tablespoons rapeseed oil

240g pearl barley

1 litre chicken stock

For the glazed beef

1 tablespoon rapeseed oil

3 fillet steaks

1 large orange, juice only

2 tablespoons maple syrup

2 tablespoons balsamic vinegar

For the dressing

small bunch fresh parsley

4 tablespoons olive oil

2 tablespoons apple cider vinegar

1 lime, juice only

1 tablespoon tahini

Preheat the oven to 180°C/350°F/gas 4.

Drizzle the olive oil over the vegetables, toss and roast for 40 minutes, until soft enough to squash between your index finger and thumb.

Meanwhile, heat the rapeseed oil in a saucepan and add the pearl barley. Cook for 3 minutes to lightly toast the grains and then add the stock and cook for 20 minutes. The pearl barley should be al dente. Remove from the heat and drain any remaining liquid.

While the pearl barley is cooking, lightly brush both sides of the steaks with the rapeseed oil and then heat a griddle pan over a medium heat. When it is hot, add the steaks, cooking until each side has browned (about 3 minutes per side). Then add the orange juice, maple syrup and balsamic vinegar, and reduce until the sauce is lovely and sticky. Remove from the heat and leave to settle while you make the dressing.

Note: For adults, if you prefer a rarer steak then cook to your own liking. Ensure the meat is fully cooked and not rare for babies.

To make the dressing, place all of the ingredients in a blender and blend until smooth. Pour over the pearl barley and toss until combined.

For babies, serve a few strips of very thinly sliced meat with a drizzle of sauce and a portion of the pearl barley and roasted vegetables on the side.

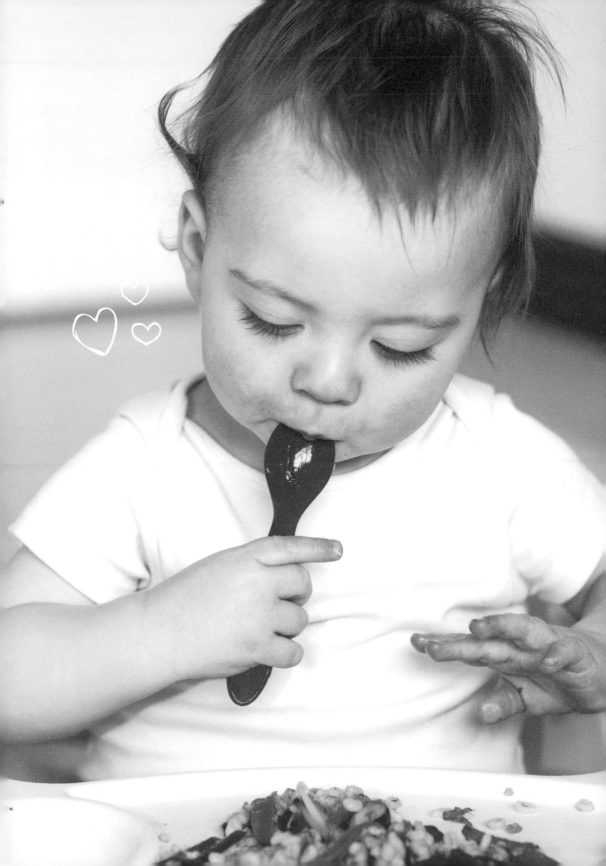

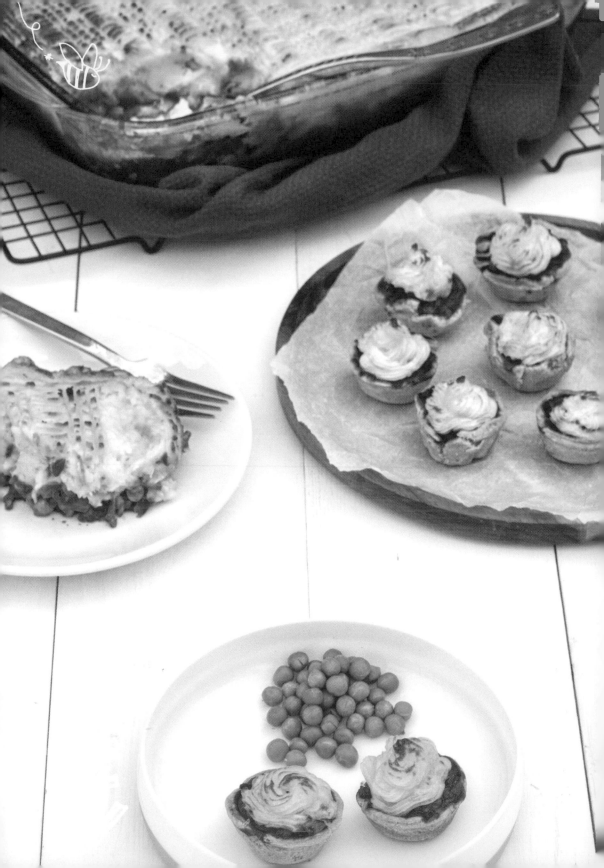

Baby Cottage Pies

Traditionally, cottage pie was a dish created to use up whatever meat and vegetables you had lying around your store cupboard or fridge, mixed with leftover gravy and topped with mashed potato, baked and served with more gravy. My healthy version, however, uses a delicious, healthy tomato gravy with lean beef and soft vegetables all topped with yogurt, olive oil and parsley mashed potatoes. My little baby found it hard to eat on his own, so for him I created little pies and piped the potato on before baking just enough to brown the spuds, making a delicious baby bite.

Serves 2 adults and 2 children, plus 24 mini-pies

For the meat sauce

4 tablespoons rapeseed oil

2 medium white onions, finely chopped

3 cloves garlic, crushed

400g lean minced beef

3 large carrots, finely chopped

2 red bell peppers, diced

3 tablespoons unsalted tomato purée

400g tinned chopped tomatoes

1 teaspoon English mustard

2 tablespoons apple cider vinegar

2 sprigs fresh thyme, leaves picked and finely chopped

pepper, to season

For the mash

2kg potatoes (Maris Piper works best), peeled and cut into chunks

60ml olive oil

80ml milk

pepper, to season

small bunch parsley, finely chopped

For the pastry

150g plain flour

80g butter

2–3 tablespoons water

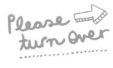
Please turn over

Heat the rapeseed oil in a saucepan over a medium heat and fry the onions until they start to turn translucent. Add the garlic and cook for another 2 minutes. Then add the minced beef and cook until it has started to brown.

Add the carrots and peppers to the pan along with the tomato purée, tinned tomatoes, mustard and vinegar. Give everything a good stir, cover the saucepan with a lid and simmer for 20 minutes until the carrots are soft enough to squash between your thumb and forefinger. Add the thyme and then season with pepper.

Take the lid off the saucepan and continue to simmer for a further 10 minutes to allow the sauce to thicken.

While the meat sauce is cooking, place the potatoes in a pot of boiling water and cook for about 20 minutes, until they are soft through, then drain.

Add the olive oil, milk, pepper and parsley and mash until smooth.

Preheat the oven to 180°C/350°F/gas 4.

Make the pastry for the mini-pies by adding the flour to a bowl and then, using your fingers, working the butter through the flour until it resembles fine breadcrumbs. Add the water one tablespoon at a time until the pastry comes together. Turn it out onto a well-floured work surface and roll until it is roughly half a centimetre thick. Cut out 24 little circles and place into a lightly oiled mini-muffin tin.

To assemble the baby cottage pies, spoon a heaped teaspoon of the meat mixture into each pastry case and add a teaspoon of mashed potato to the top of each one. (I use a piping bag for cuteness.)

Pour the remaining meat mixture into a deep baking dish and top with the potato. Flatten with the back of a spoon to make sure the meat is totally covered. Use the prongs of a fork to decorate the top.

Place the mini pies and the large pie in the oven and bake for 25 minutes. The top of the potato should be golden brown.

Cool slightly before serving.

Fish Pies
with Steamed Broccoli

Deliciously creamy fish pies, perfect for cold and dreary winters when you are looking for comforting and nutritious food.

Serves 2 adults and 2 children

For the topping

2kg potatoes (Maris Piper works best), peeled and washed

60ml olive oil

80ml milk

pepper, to season

small bunch parsley, finely chopped

For the filling

3 tablespoons rapeseed oil

1 large white onion, finely chopped

4 cloves garlic, crushed

150ml fresh cream

100g frozen garden peas

small bunch fresh chives, finely chopped

small bunch parsley, finely chopped

½ teaspoon Dijon mustard

700g fresh fish of your choice, cut into chunks

150ml natural yogurt

½ lemon, juice only

2 large handfuls baby leaf spinach, finely chopped

Preheat oven to 180°/350°F/gas 4.

To make the topping, peel and wash the potatoes, then add to a saucepan and cover with water. Bring to the boil, cover and simmer for about 25 minutes until the potatoes are soft, then drain.

Add the oil, milk, pepper and parsley to the potatoes and mash until smooth and creamy, then set aside.

To make the filling, heat oil in a pan over a medium heat and fry the onion until it is starting to turn golden. This takes about 6 minutes. Add the garlic and cook for a further 2 minutes until lovely and fragrant.

Turn the heat to low and then add the cream along with the frozen peas, chives, parsley and mustard.

Check there are no bones left in the fish, then add to the pot and simmer for about 10 minutes until the fish is cooked. Remove from the heat and stir in the yogurt, lemon juice and spinach. Give everything a good stir, then pour into an ovenproof dish.

Spoon the mashed potato over the fish and smooth down with the back of a spoon. Using a fork, draw lines across the potato to decorate.

Bake for 30 minutes.

Serve warm.

Chicken & Broccoli
Baby Pies

OK, hands up – I admit I am a huge fan of pies, pie with mash and peas being my ultimate comfort dish when I've had a hard day, and my love of pies has fortunately passed on to my entire family. Mini-pies are brilliant for little hands and you can pack them with whatever good stuff you have cooking.

Makes 12 large and 24 mini-pies

For the filling

2 tablespoons rapeseed oil

2 medium white onions, finely chopped

4 free-range chicken breasts, cut into small pieces

3 cloves garlic, crushed

120g broccoli, finely chopped

80g frozen garden peas

160ml fresh cream

80ml natural yogurt

1 teaspoon Dijon mustard

pepper, to season

For the pastry

450g plain flour

240g butter

8 tablespoons water

1 egg, beaten, for brushing

Preheat the oven to 180°C/350°F/gas 4.

Heat the rapeseed oil in a frying pan over a medium heat and fry the onions for about 3 minutes, until they start to turn translucent. Add the chicken to the pan and cook for about 10 minutes until the chicken is cooked through. Add the garlic and broccoli along with the frozen peas.

Next add the cream, yogurt, mustard and pepper, give everything a good stir, then simmer for about 20 minutes.

Meanwhile, make the pastry by adding the flour to a bowl and then, using your fingers, working the butter through until it resembles fine breadcrumbs. Add the water one tablespoon at a time until the pastry comes together. Turn it out onto a well-floured work surface and cut in half. Roll one of the dough halves until it is roughly half a centimetre thick, then cut out 24 little circles to fit a mini-muffin tin and 12 to fit a standard muffin tin. Lightly oil the tins and place a pastry circle in each cup.

When the meat mixture is cooked, use it to fill each pastry case up to the top. Roll out the other half of the pastry, cut out lids to fit the pies and place them on top.

Brush a little beaten egg on each pastry lid and then bake for 25 minutes until the pastry is golden brown.

Serve warm.

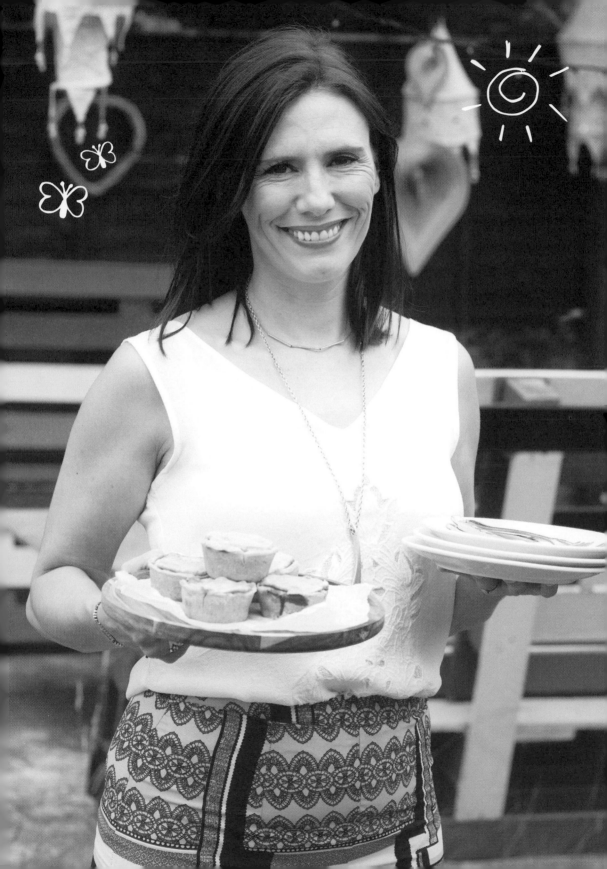

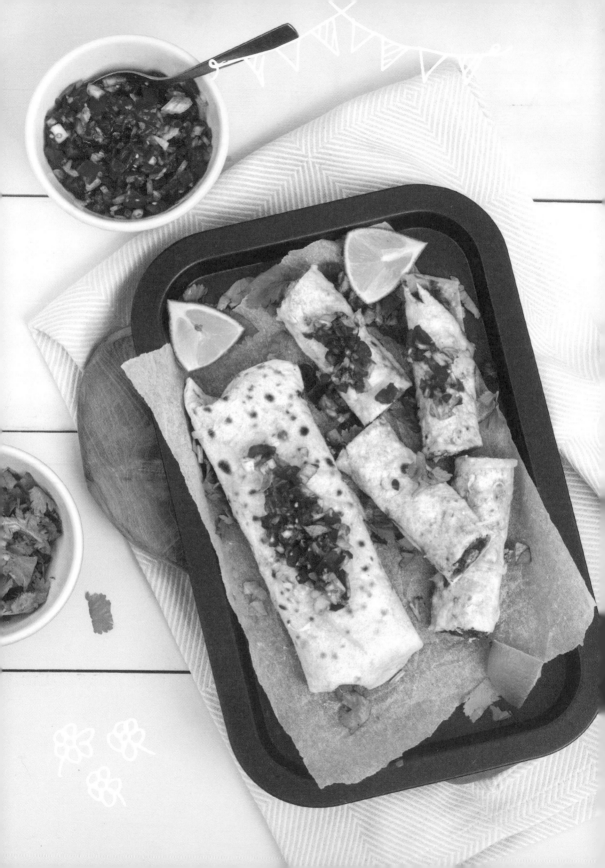

Mexican Taquitos with Pulled Pork

Taquitos are like a very skinny burrito – a flour tortilla filled with beans, cheese and meat, then rolled and usually fried. These ones, however, are baked for just long enough to hold the tortilla together, making them the least messy way ever to get your little one eating Mexican food.

Makes 4 baby-sized taquitos and 4 burritos

2 tablespoons rapeseed or olive oil

320g lean diced pork

2 medium white onions, finely chopped

1 red bell pepper, finely diced

1 lime, juice only

1 teaspoon ground cumin

1 teaspoon ground coriander

1 teaspoon cinnamon

2 teaspoons paprika

½ teaspoon mild chilli powder (optional)

400g tinned tomatoes

3 tablespoons unsalted tomato purée

1 tablespoon apple cider vinegar

pepper, to season

400g tin black beans or kidney beans, drained

small bunch fresh coriander

50g cheddar cheese

4 x 15cm and 4 x 30cm tortillas (see page 143)

Preheat oven to 160°C/325°F/gas 3.

Heat the oil in a frying pan, add the pork and cook over a very low heat. Add the vegetables to the pan along with the lime juice, spices, tin of tomatoes, tomato purée, vinegar and pepper. Cover the pot with a lid and slow cook for 2 hours until the meat becomes tender. Add the beans for the last 20 minutes of cooking and remove the lid to allow the sauce to thicken.

To assemble each taquito, take a heaped tablespoon of the meat and vegetable mixture and spread lengthways across the middle of a 15cm tortilla, sprinkle over a little cheddar cheese and roll into a tight log shape. Place on a baking tray lightly oiled with rapeseed oil. When all the taquitos are rolled, sprinkle a little extra cheese on top and bake for 12 minutes, until the cheese starts to melt and the tortillas are stuck together. Cool slightly before serving.

Assemble the burritos in the same way, but add more of the mixture for older children and grown-ups. Top with a little salsa or homemade guacamole (see page 201).

Baby Veggie Burgers

As vegetarian burgers go, these are the best I have tasted. They aren't dry or tasteless like so many I have tried over the years, and they have a firm texture which makes it easy for little ones to manage.

Makes 8 mini-burgers and 4 large burgers

For the burgers

1 medium onion, finely chopped

2 cloves garlic, crushed

60g uncooked red lentils

60g uncooked green lentils

100g brown rice

140g peas

140g sweetcorn

400g tin kidney beans, drained

2 tablespoons flaxseed

¼ teaspoon ground cumin

¼ teaspoon dried coriander

¼ teaspoon mild chilli powder

80g breadcrumbs

30g fresh coriander, finely chopped

pepper, to season

2 eggs

rapeseed oil, for frying

Pull & Share White Bread Rolls (see page 66)

Heat a little oil in a frying pan. Add the onion and sauté for about 3 minutes, until soft. Add the garlic and cook for another 2 minutes until soft but not browned.

Place the lentils, the rice and the remaining ingredients, except the eggs, in a bowl and mix well. Whisk the eggs in a separate bowl and then add to the rest of the ingredients. This will help bind the mixture.

Take a couple of tablespoons of the mixture and, using your hands, shape into a baby-sized veggie burger. Repeat until you have 8 burgers. Then divide the remaining mixture into 4 and shape these into larger burgers.

To cook the burgers, heat about 1 tablespoon of rapeseed oil per batch in a frying pan over a medium heat. Place a few burgers on the pan and cook for about 4 minutes. Then flip them over and cook for a further 4 minutes the other side. They should be lovely and golden brown.

To serve, place each burger in a roll, top with a little thinly sliced sweet onion, sliced tomato and some Cajun Sauce (page 204). Add some potato wedges on the side.

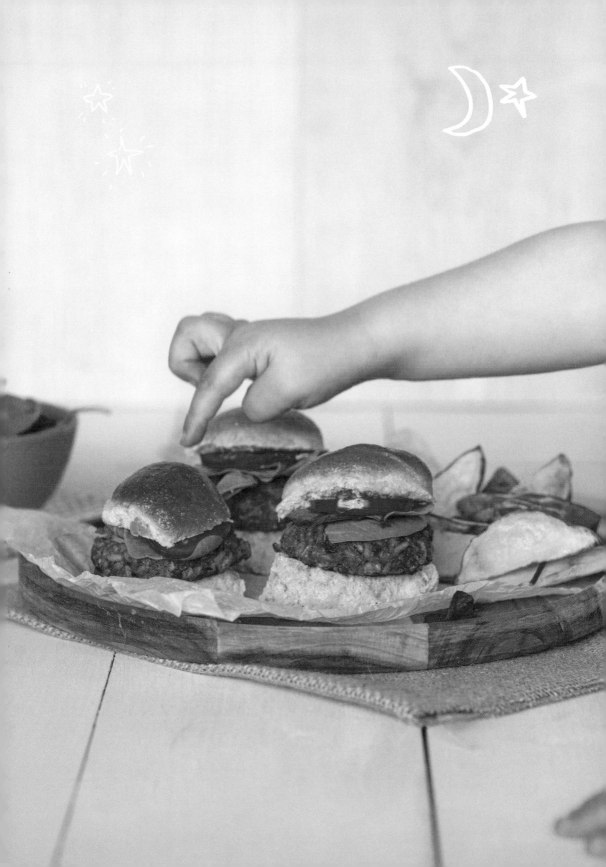

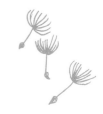

Beef Burgers
with Roasted Veggie Chips

Burgers are a great way to get your little ones to eat red meat. They are also a great way to get kids eating vegetables. The baby sees the older kids eating burgers with a little lettuce, tomato and onion and wants to have his burger just like them. He may end up eating everything separately until he gets the hang of holding it all together in a bun, but that's all part of the fun of learning.

Makes 2 baby-, 2 kid- and 2 adult-sized burgers

For the chips

2 large sweet potatoes, peeled and cut into chips

1 parsnip, peeled and cut into chips

2 beetroot, peeled and cut into chips

sprig of fresh rosemary, leaves picked and finely chopped

2 tablespoons rapeseed oil

1 teaspoon paprika

For the burgers

380g lean minced beef

1 egg

60g breadcrumbs

1 teaspoon Dijon mustard

pepper, to season

To serve

Pull & Share White Bread Rolls (see page 66)

Preheat oven to 180°C/350°F/gas 4.

Place the sweet potato, parsnip and beetroot into a bowl. Add the rosemary, oil and paprika. Use your hands to make sure everything is completely coated. Then place the chips on a tray lined with parchment paper. Roast for 35 minutes.

While the vegetables are cooking, make the burgers by adding all of the ingredients to a large bowl and, using your hands again, mixing well.

Divide the meat into 4 parts. Shape 2 parts into large burgers for the adults. Remove a small piece from each of the remaining 2 parts and shape into baby-sized burgers. Shape what's left into 2 burgers for the older kids. To cook the burgers, heat about 1 tablespoon of rapeseed oil per batch in a frying pan over a medium heat. Place a few burgers on the pan and cook for about 4–5 minutes on each side. They should be golden brown and cooked through.

Pull off a bread roll for each burger. Gently toast the bread and place a burger on top. Garnish with some thinly sliced tomato and onion, shredded lettuce and a little Baby Ketchup (see page 203). Serve with the softly roasted veggie chips.

Moroccan Chicken

with Roasted Vegetables & Mint Yogurt Dressing

Warm, fragrant chicken coated in Moroccan spices and served with soft roasted vegetables and a mint yogurt dressing – it sounds fancy but takes less than 15 minutes to prepare and cooks away in the oven while you spend time playing with your family.

Serves 2 adults and 2 children

For the chicken

1 whole chicken, quartered

1 heaped teaspoon ground cumin

1 heaped teaspoon paprika

1 heaped teaspoon ground coriander

1 heaped teaspoon ground ginger

1 heaped teaspoon dried thyme

3 tablespoons rapeseed oil

2 tablespoons apple cider vinegar

thumb-sized piece root ginger, grated

For the vegetables

1 large onion, roughly chopped

2 red peppers, chopped into large chunks

1 courgette, chopped into large chunks

2 large sweet potatoes, scrubbed and chopped into large chunks

drizzle of olive oil

4 cloves garlic, skin on

For the sauce

roasted garlic (see vegetables)

125ml natural yogurt

1 lime, zest of whole lime and juice of ½

handful mint leaves, finely chopped

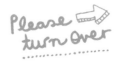

Please turn over

Preheat oven to 170°C/325°F/gas 3.

Place the quartered chicken into a baking dish and use a sharp knife to stab holes in it so that the sauce can get to all parts of the meat.

Mix all of the remaining ingredients for the chicken in a bowl. Pour over the chicken, then, using your hands, massage into the meat, making sure all parts of the chicken are covered.

Place the chicken in the oven and bake for 1 hour, ensuring the legs are fully cooked before removing – when a skewer is inserted in the thickest part of the leg, the juices should run clear.

Meanwhile, place the vegetables on a baking tray and drizzle with the oil. Use your hands to make sure all the vegetables are well covered. Scatter the cloves of garlic through the vegetables. You will be using these later for the yogurt sauce.

When the chicken has been baking for 20 minutes, add the vegetables to the oven. The vegetables should take about 40 minutes to cook through.

When cooked, take the vegetables and the chicken out of the oven. Remove the garlic cloves from the vegetables, peel them and add the flesh to a bowl. Mash well and add the yogurt, lime zest, juice and the mint. Give it all a good mix.

Cut some soft pieces of chicken, making sure there are no bones, for the baby. Add a few pieces of sweet potato and veg and top with some yogurt sauce.

For the grown-ups, just place the chicken on a large platter and surround with the vegetables. Serve the yogurt sauce in a bowl and let everyone help themselves.

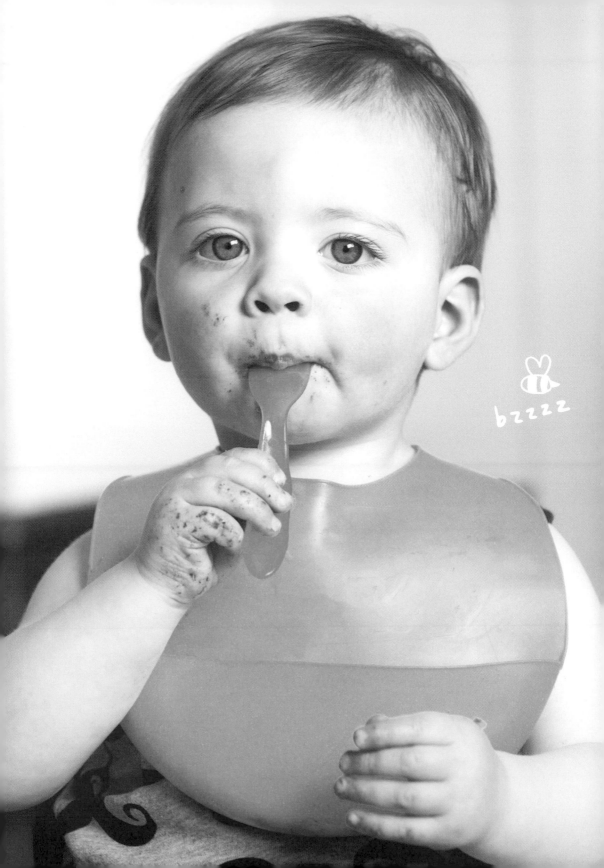
bzzzz

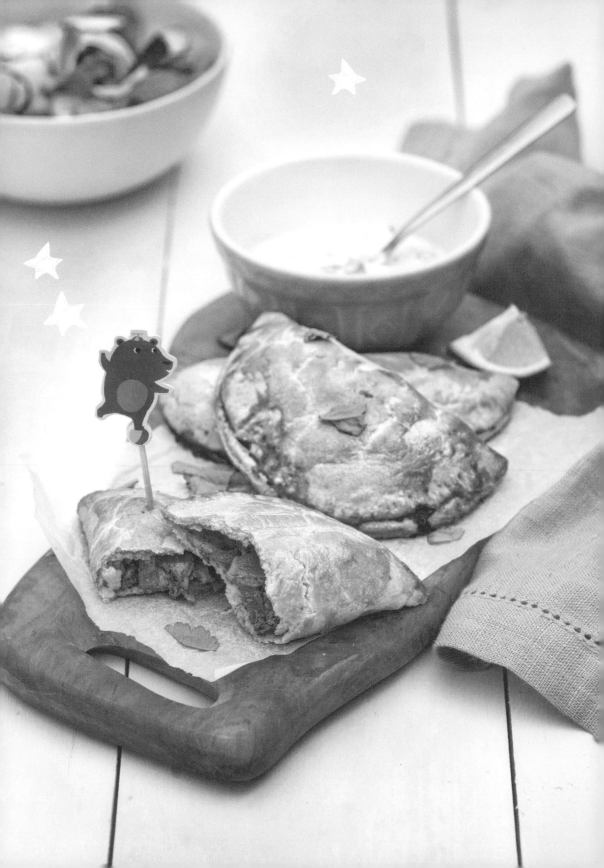

Lamb Shawarma Pasties

This is probably one of my favourite ways to eat lamb – slowly cooked to ensure it is tender enough for the smallest of weaning babies, bursting with aromatic Middle Eastern spices and served with a delicious tzatziki. For the baby, I make a batch of little pasties filled with the lamb mixture and baked to make it easier for them to eat.

Serves 2 adults and 2 children

For the shawarma

280g lean diced lamb

2 tablespoons rapeseed oil

1 teaspoon ground cumin

1 teaspoon ground coriander

1 teaspoon cinnamon

1 teaspoon paprika

1 teaspoon ground ginger

1 teaspoon turmeric

4 cardamom pods, seeds only

400g tinned tomatoes

100ml water

pepper, to season

For the pastry

300g plain flour

150g butter

4 tablespoons water

1 egg, beaten

For the tzatziki

120ml natural yogurt

2 cloves roasted garlic, crushed

½ lemon, juice only

160g cucumber, peeled and finely chopped

pepper, to season

In a saucepan, fry the lamb in the oil to seal the meat. Add the remaining ingredients for the shawarma to the pan and stir until totally combined.

Cook on the lowest heat for 4–5 hours so that the lamb is tender and soft. I use a slow cooker on its medium setting for 4 hours. Remove the lid for the last 30 minutes to allow the sauce to thicken up.

Preheat oven to 180°C/350°F/gas 4.

To make the pastry, sieve the flour into a bowl and, using your fingers, work the butter in until the mixture starts to resemble fine breadcrumbs. Add the water a tablespoon at a time until the pastry comes together. Wrap the pastry in cling film and place in the refrigerator until you are ready to assemble the pasties.

Place the pastry onto a lightly floured surface and roll until about half a centimetre thick. Cut out 10 circles, each roughly measuring 10cm.

Take a heaped tablespoon of the shawarma and place into the centre of each pastry circle. Brush a little beaten egg around the edges before folding in half and pressing the two sides together to seal. Make 2 small holes in the top of each pasty, brush with the remaining egg wash and place on a lightly oiled baking tray. Bake for 25 minutes, until the pastry is golden brown.

Make the tzatziki by adding all of the ingredients to a bowl and stirring well. Serve each pasty with a dollop of sauce on the side.

Little Baby BUDDHA Bowls

Blue Bowl

Roasted sweet potato with stir-fried spinach, roasted chickpeas, avocado and sour cream.

A Buddha Bowl sounds like some sort of religious ritual, but it is just a fancy name for a bowl full of simple, pure food that is enjoyed with a smile.

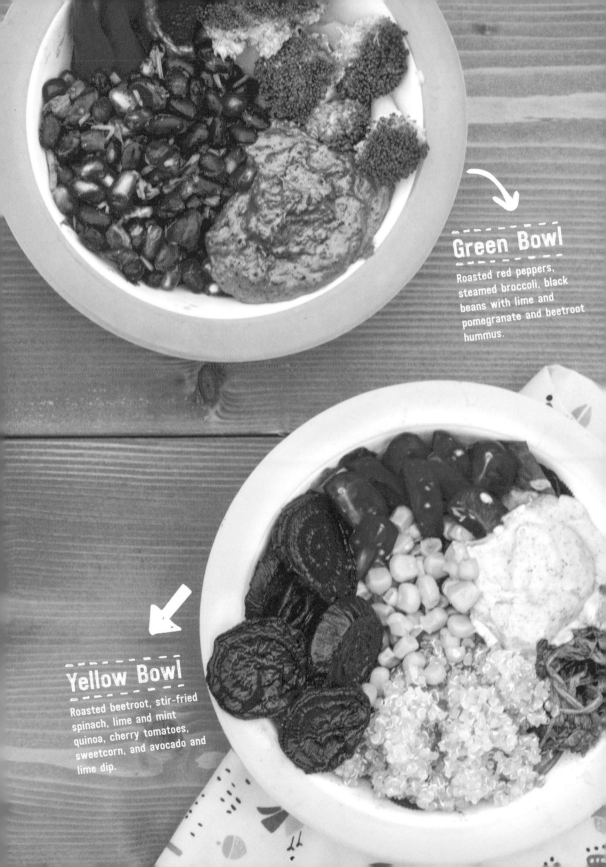

Green Bowl

Roasted red peppers, steamed broccoli, black beans with lime and pomegranate and beetroot hummus.

Yellow Bowl

Roasted beetroot, stir-fried spinach, lime and mint quinoa, cherry tomatoes, sweetcorn, and avocado and lime dip.

What Goes into
a Buddha Bowl

These bowls of goodness can be made with whatever ingredients you have in your refrigerator, once they have a good balance of nutrients. I like to make mine in thirds: one-third protein (meat, fish, beans etc.), one-third grains or legumes (couscous, quinoa, chickpeas, beans) and one-third vegetables. This is all topped off with a sauce or dip of your choice. These are some of my favourite things to include – all baby friendly and so quick to make. They also look deliciously colourful and are guaranteed to make you smile.

Serves 2 adults and 2 kids

Lime and Mint Quinoa

70g quinoa
160ml water
1 tablespoon olive oil
1 lime, juice and zest
10 mint leaves, finely chopped

Add the quinoa and water to a saucepan and bring to the boil. Reduce the heat to a simmer, cover with a lid and cook for 15 minutes, until the water has been completely absorbed and the quinoa is cooked.

In the meantime, make the dressing by adding the remaining ingredients to a bowl and mixing well.

When the quinoa is cooked, pour the dressing on top and stir through.

Serve warm.

Roasted Chickpeas

400g tinned chickpeas, drained
drizzle of olive oil
½ teaspoon paprika
½ teaspoon ground coriander
½ teaspoon ground cumin

Preheat oven to 180°C/350°F/gas 4.

Place all the ingredients in a bowl. Mix well and place on a baking sheet lined with parchment paper.

Roast for just 25 minutes – they should still be soft for little mouths.

Before serving to babies, lightly crush the chickpeas.

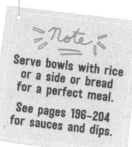

Note

Serve bowls with rice or a side or bread for a perfect meal.

See pages 196-204 for sauces and dips.

Stir-Fried Spinach

1 tablespoon olive oil

1 clove garlic, crushed

1 tablespoon water

2 large handfuls spinach, roughly chopped

Heat the olive oil in a frying pan over a medium heat. Add the garlic and fry for 2 minutes, making sure not to burn it.

Add the water to the pan then add the spinach leaves and cook for about 1 minute, until they are just starting to wilt.

Serve warm.

Roasted Beetroot

1 medium-sized beetroot

2 tablespoons coconut oil, melted

Preheat oven to 180°C/350°F/gas 4.

Cut the beetroot into thin strips, place onto kitchen foil then pour over the coconut oil. Fold the foil into a parcel, seal and place in the oven. Bake for around 40 minutes, until the beetroot is soft enough to be squashed between your index finger and thumb.

Avocado and Lime Dip

1 avocado

½ lime, juice only

small bunch fresh coriander

2 cloves roasted garlic

Place all of the ingredients in a food processor and blend until the sauce becomes smooth and creamy.

Black Beans with Lime and Pomegranate

400g tinned black beans, drained

1 lime, juice only

½ pomegranate, seeds only

small bunch fresh coriander, finely chopped

Add all the ingredients to a bowl and stir well.

Beetroot Hummus

6 cloves garlic, roasted

400g tinned chickpeas

4 tablespoons tahini

4 tablespoons extra virgin olive oil

4 tablespoons water

1 lemon, juice only

1 cooked medium beetroot

Add all of the ingredients to a food processor and process until the hummus is deliciously creamy.

Egg Roulade
with Spinach and Goat's Cheese Filling

My mother taught me how to make roulades when I was a kid and I have made
many over the years, sweet and savoury, which have all been delicious, light and
fluffy. This roulade is great for babies, as not only is it easy to pick up but the
ingredients are also nutritious and healthy, and it looks fancy enough to serve to
Nana for Sunday brunch.

Serves 2 adults and 2 children

80g unsalted butter

4 tablespoons plain flour

400ml milk

4 eggs, separated

1 tablespoon olive oil

1 medium white onion,
finely chopped

2 cloves garlic, crushed

80g spinach, roughly
chopped

120ml natural yogurt

90g goat's cheese

1 teaspoon Dijon mustard

2 sprigs fresh thyme, leaves
picked and finely chopped

Preheat oven to 200°C/400°F/gas 6.

In a saucepan, gently melt the butter. Add the flour and,
using a whisk, stir well to make a roux. Very slowly pour
in the milk, whisking all the while to prevent lumps. You
should be left with a thick white sauce. Remove from the
heat, add the egg yolks and stir well to make sure they are
fully combined.

In a separate bowl, whisk the egg whites until light and
fluffy and forming peaks. Then, using a spatula, fold the egg
whites into the white sauce.

Line a 38 x 26cm baking tin with parchment paper, then
pour the egg mixture onto it. Use the spatula to make sure
it is evenly spread. Bake for 15 minutes until the egg is fully
set. Then leave aside to cool.

In the meantime, heat the olive oil in a pan over a medium
heat. Gently fry the onion until golden and sticky – this
should take about 8 minutes. Add the garlic and cook for
another 2 minutes. Next add the spinach, yogurt, goat's
cheese, mustard and thyme. Stir until the cheese has fully
melted then remove from the heat.

When the egg sheet has fully cooled, flip it over and gently
remove the parchment paper. Spoon the spinach and
yogurt filling on top and spread all over before rolling up
into a roulade shape. Serve immediately.

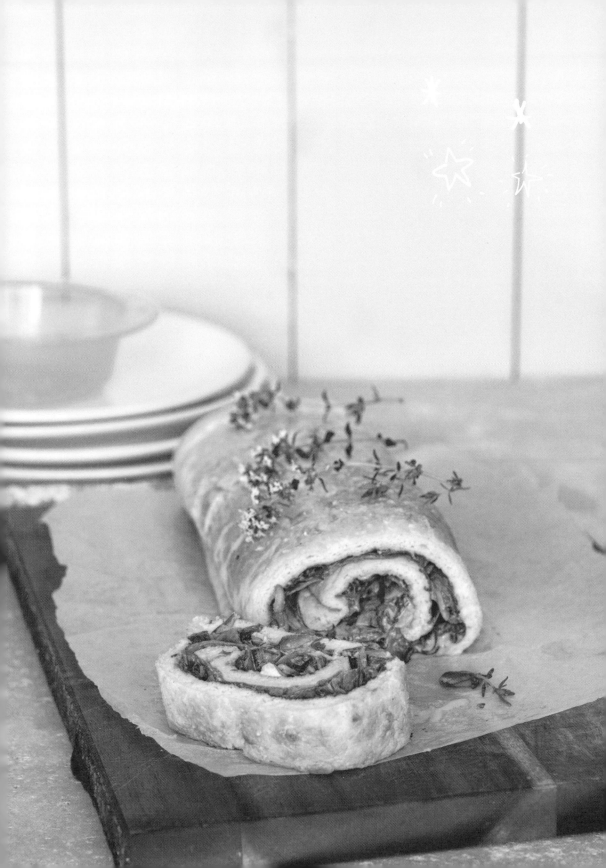

Rice-Paper Rolls
with Pork

After seeing what looked like a very simple video on how to make your own rice paper, I gave it a shot – and failed miserably. It was much harder than it looked, so I went to my local Asian store and bought a great value pack of organic rice paper that contained just two ingredients: rice and semolina flour. Happy with my purchase, I went home and made these little rolls, which were delicious. It is essentially a pork stir-fry in a wrap, which makes it really easy for babies' hands, and it's very nutritious.

Makes 12 rolls

200g carrot, cut into long, thin sticks

2 tablespoons rapeseed or olive oil

200g free range pork, finely diced

100g white onion, finely sliced

15g root ginger, grated

80g sprouted lentils

150g beansprouts

2 tablespoons apple cider vinegar

1 tablespoon natural fish sauce

12 basil leaves, finely chopped

12 rice paper rolls

Steam the carrots for about 20 minutes, until you are able to squash them between your forefinger and thumb.

Heat the oil over a medium-to-low heat and gently fry the pork until cooked through. Add the onion and cook for a further 3 minutes, until it starts to turn translucent. Then add the grated ginger, sprouted lentils and beansprouts and cook just enough to heat through.

Stir in the apple cider vinegar and fish sauce, and then remove the pan from the heat. Add the basil leaves and give everything a good stir.

To make the rolls, fill a large bowl three-quarter's full of warm water. Place each sheet of rice paper into the bowl for 3 seconds. It will still be firm when you take it out but will continue to soften while you add the filling.

Put the rice paper on a plate and place a heaped tablespoon of the meat mixture in the middle. Add a few sticks of carrot and then, using your fingers, roll tightly, tucking under the sides as you do. Repeat for all 12 rolls.

Serve warm with Toddler-Friendly Asian Dip (see page 204).

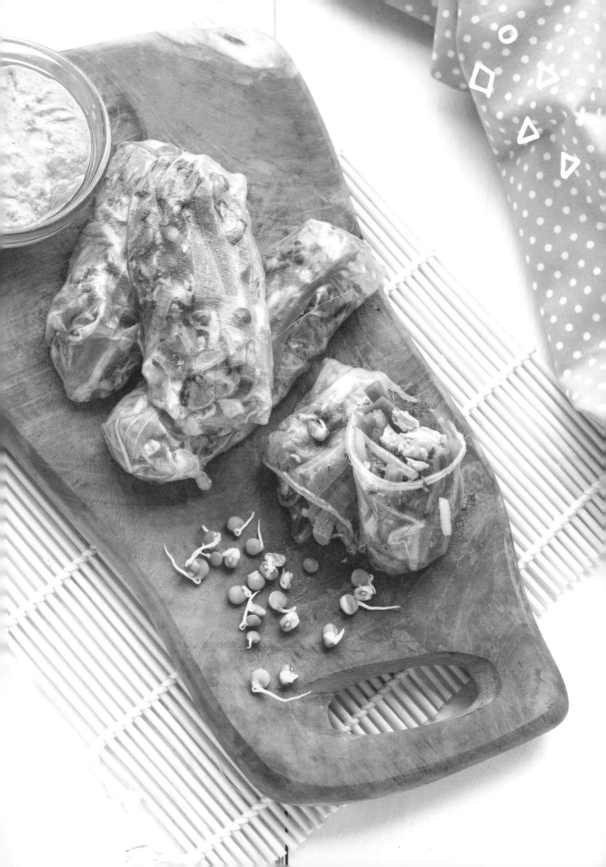

Baby Sushi Rolls

I love sushi! I would happily eat it every day, and so when I discovered my daughter was a sushi lover too I was in heaven. We learnt how to make it home, as it was much cheaper, but now that my little baby is trying to grab everything off my plate, I wanted to make a baby-friendly sushi just for him. He loves these little rolls filled with cooked fish and some veggie ones on the side.

Makes 24 pieces

For the sushi

200g sushi rice

500ml water

1 tablespoon apple cider vinegar

5 sheets nori seaweed

1 cucumber, cut in half lengthways

1 avocado, sliced

140g cooked crabmeat

80g cooked prawns, finely chopped

2 tablespoons goat's cheese

1 medium-sized carrot, steamed and cut into sticks

2 long-stem pieces broccoli, steamed and cut into sticks

For the dipping sauce

2 tablespoons apple cider vinegar

2 tablespoons natural fish sauce

½ lime, juice only

½ teaspoon wasabi powder (optional)

Place the rice in a pot with the water, bring to the boil and cook for 10 minutes until the rice is soft and tender. Remove from the heat, stir in the vinegar and leave aside to fully cool.

To make the sushi, cover a sushi mat with cling film. Place a sheet of nori rough-side down on the film. Keep a bowl of water beside you and wet your hands before spreading the rice all over the seaweed.

Peel one of the cucumber halves and cut into fingers. Place strips of cucumber, avocado and either crabmeat or prawns across the middle of the seaweed. Then lightly wet your hands and, using the sushi mat, with your fingers underneath, roll the front of the nori over the filling. Tightly squeeze with your hand and then, rocking it over and back, shape into a tight roll.

Wet a sharp knife and cut the roll into 8 even pieces. To do this, I cut a roll in half, then place the halves beside each other, cut in half again and repeat. Wrap in cling film and store in the fridge until you are ready to serve.

To make vegetarian sushi, take the other cucumber half and, using a vegetable peeler, peel long strips and lay them out flat. Spoon a little goat's cheese along a quarter of each cucumber strip, add a few soft carrot sticks and a little broccoli and roll into a sushi shape.

To make the dip, combine all the ingredients in a bowl and mix well. Serve the sushi fresh with dipping sauce on the side.

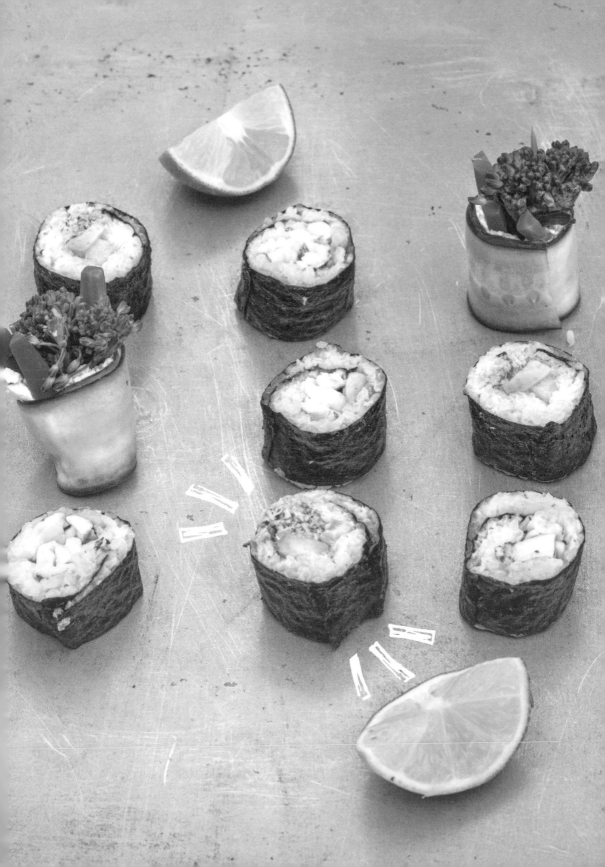

Baked Avocados with Roasted Tomato Sauce & Black Beans

Avocados are an all-round amazing food, full of heart-healthy fats and incredibly nutritious. If you are a fan but have only eaten them in guacamole or salad then this is the dish for you (and your little ones). Baking avocados makes them even creamier, and then you just add an egg, some tomato sauce and black beans to make a perfect weekend brunch or dinner.

Serves 2

1 avocado

2 eggs

drizzle olive oil

For the roasted tomato sauce

24 cherry tomatoes

8 cloves garlic (skin on)

1 tablespoon apple cider vinegar

2 tablespoons tomato purée

1 teaspoon Dijon mustard

12 basil leaves

60ml water

1 quantity Black Beans with Lime and Pomegranate (see page 173), warmed

small bunch fresh coriander, finely chopped

Preheat oven to 180°C/350°F/gas 4.

Cut the avocado in half and take the stone out. Scoop a little avocado out of each half to make a bigger dip for the egg. Place the avocado halves on a baking sheet lined with parchment paper.

Crack one egg into each half of the avocado, drizzle with olive oil and bake for 20 minutes until the egg is cooked through and set.

To make the roasted tomato sauce, place the tomatoes and garlic on a baking tray and bake for 20 minutes (do this at the same time as you cook the avocados).

When the tomatoes and garlic are cooked, remove the skin from the garlic, add all of the ingredients to a blender and blend until smooth.

To serve, place each avocado half on a plate along with some beans and drizzle over some tomato sauce. Sprinkle with a little extra coriander to make it look pretty. For babies, peel the avocado, chop it and the egg into chunks and serve.

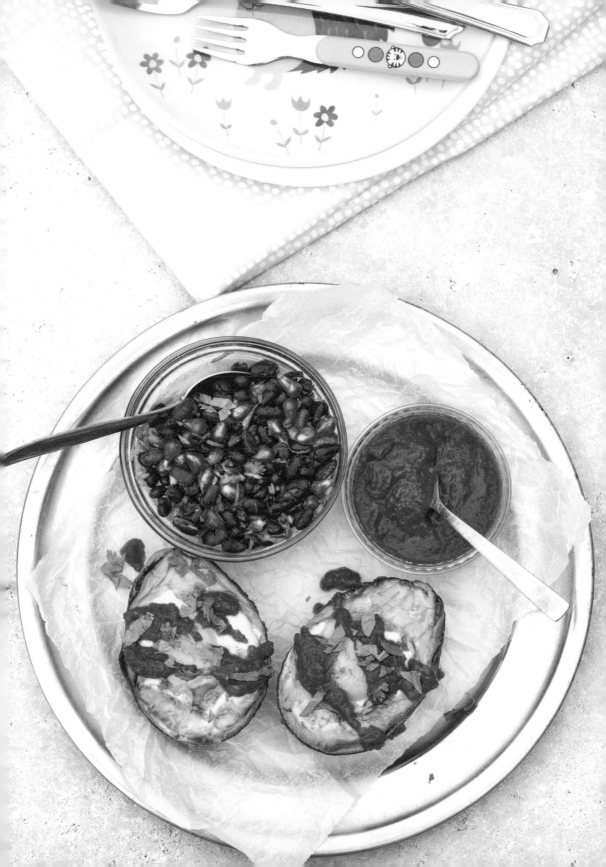

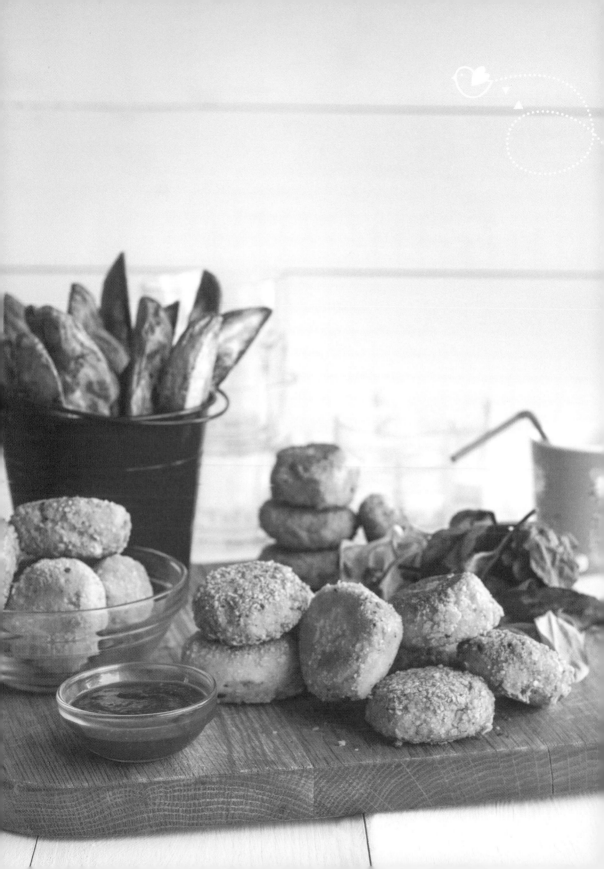

Healthy Chicken Nuggets with Potato Wedges

One of the reasons processed chicken nuggets are so popular with kids is because of their size – they are easy and manageable to eat. However, they are also high in salt, fat and other not-so-nice ingredients, so I decided to make my own more nutritious version. These are an all-round winner for kids. They are made using soft chicken breast blended with oats, egg and garlic and then coated in breadcrumbs and baked. Super healthy and super yum!

Serves 2 adults and 2 children

2 large potatoes, scrubbed and cut into spears

olive oil, for drizzling

2 cooked free-range chicken breasts

4 tablespoons oats

2 eggs

4 cloves garlic, roasted

1 teaspoon onion powder

100g breadcrumbs

60g ground almonds (optional)

black pepper, to season

Preheat oven to 180°C/350°F/gas 4.

Place the potatoes into a large bowl, drizzle with olive oil, then bake in the oven for about 30 minutes.

While the potato is cooking, place the chicken breasts and oats into a food processor and blend until it's the texture of fine breadcrumbs.

Scoop the mixture into a bowl, add one egg, the garlic and the onion powder and give it a good stir to totally combine.

In a separate bowl, whisk the remaining egg. In an additional bowl, add the breadcrumbs, ground almonds (if using) and black pepper.

Shape the chicken mixture into small bite-sized pieces, then dip each one into the beaten egg and coat in breadcrumbs.

Place on an oiled baking tray and bake for 10 minutes. Flip them over and bake for a further 10 minutes.

Serve with the potato wedges and Baby Ketchup (see page 203).

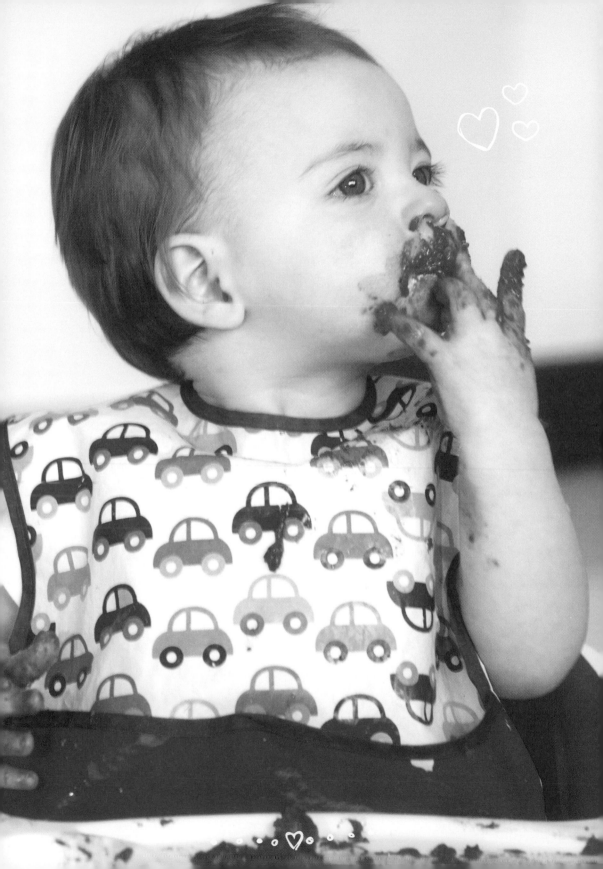

Turkey Meatballs

Watching my six-month-old tucking into turkey meatballs covered in a rich tomato sauce and layered on top of some spaghetti is still, to this day, the funniest memory I have of him weaning. Meatballs are a great size for little hands and the sauce clings to the spaghetti, making it really easy for them to handle.

Serves 2 adults and 2 children

For the meatballs

1 small onion, finely diced

rapeseed or olive oil, for frying

1 clove garlic

500g minced turkey

30g breadcrumbs

2 heaped tablespoons hard goat's cheese, grated

1 egg

½ teaspoon ground black pepper

For the sauce

1 tablespoon rapeseed or olive oil

1 small white onion, finely chopped

1 red bell pepper, finely chopped

1 tablespoon unsalted tomato purée

400g tinned tomatoes

2 teaspoons apple cider vinegar

¼ teaspoon English mustard

125ml milk of your choice

10 leaves fresh basil, finely chopped

To make the meatballs, gently fry the onion in a little olive or rapeseed oil until it is nice and soft. Add the garlic and cook for another 2–3 minutes over a medium heat.

When cooked, add to a mixing bowl along with the remaining meatball ingredients and mix really well.

Take about a tablespoon of the mixture and, using your hands, roll into little meatballs about the size of a cherry tomato.

When you are finished, put all the meatballs on a plate, cover with cling film and place into the fridge for about half an hour while you make your sauce.

Heat the oil in a saucepan over a medium heat and gently fry the onion and pepper until soft. This should take about 8 minutes. Add the tomato purée, tinned tomatoes, apple cider vinegar and mustard and stir really well.

Pour the mixture into a blender and whizz up until really smooth. Then pour back into the saucepan. Add the milk, stir well and cook until the sauce starts to bubble. Then turn the heat down to a simmer.

Add the meatballs to the sauce. It's important not to stir them so that they don't break up (lesson learnt the hard way!). Cover the saucepan and leave to simmer for about 20 minutes or until the meatballs are cooked through. You can take one out and check it by cutting in half.

Serve with the pasta of your choice – my little one loves spaghetti – and some basil sprinkled on top.

Finger-Lickin' Dips & Sauces

It is really easy to reach for store-bought

sauces and dips

but these recipes are not only simple to make:
they also taste so much better. Bursting with
healthy goodness that will nourish
your entire family, they make the perfect baby
snack or side for your favourite dish.

Banana Custard

This is a deliciously creamy custard that tastes gorgeous when poured over fresh fruit or mince pies – or even eaten on its own. It is quick to make and uses only bananas to sweeten.

Serves 2 adults and 2 children

250ml milk

125ml double cream

2 bananas, peeled

1 egg yolk

1 teaspoon vanilla extract

2 teaspoons cornflour

Add the milk, cream and bananas to a blender and blend until smooth and silky. Then pour into a saucepan. Heat slowly, stirring often and being careful not to allow it to boil. When the milk and cream are hot, remove the saucepan from the heat and leave aside.

In a bowl, beat the egg yolk and vanilla until creamy and then mix in the cornflour until fully combined.

Pour about half of the milk and cream mixture into the egg bowl, whisking as you do. This will prevent the egg from curdling. Give it a good stir and then pour it all back into the saucepan and place over a low heat. Stir well until it thickens up.

Remove from the heat and serve warm over fruit or pies or just eat from the bowl.

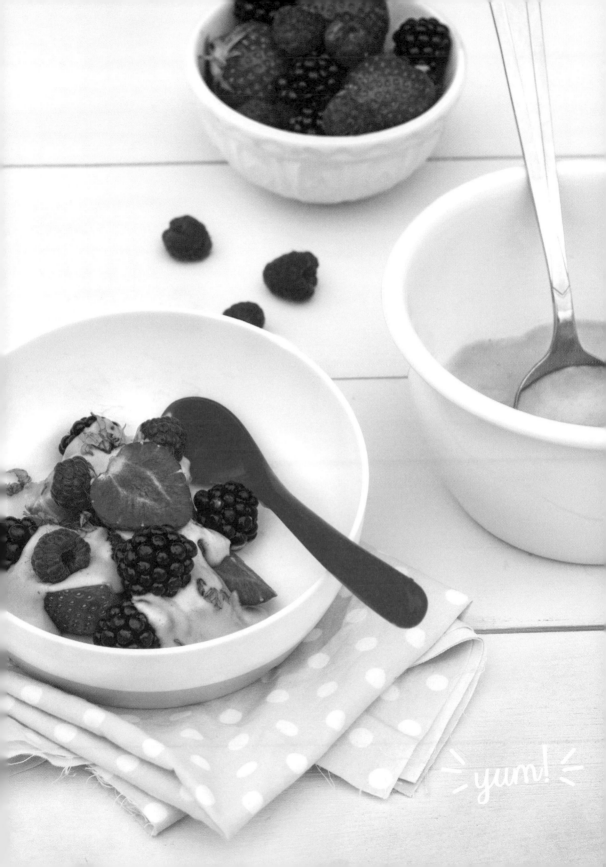

yum!

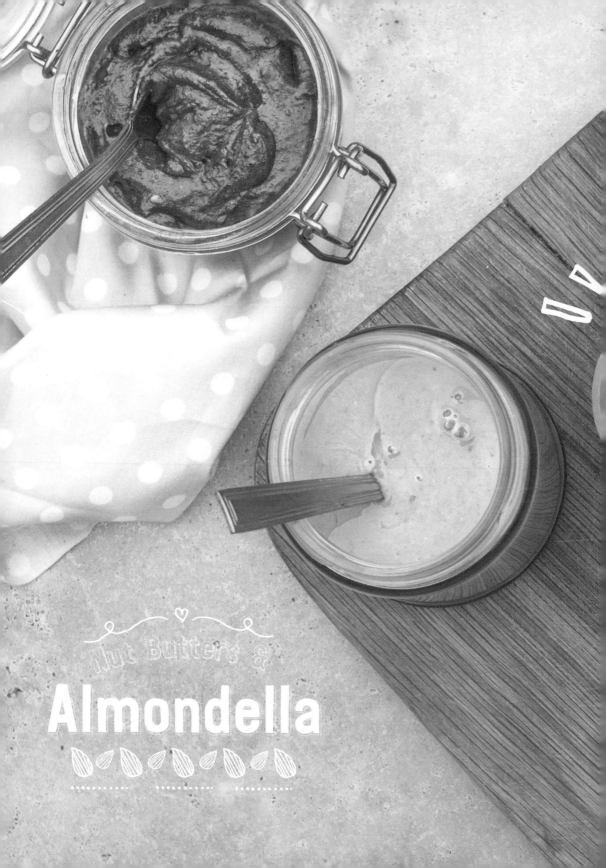

Nut Butters &

Almondella

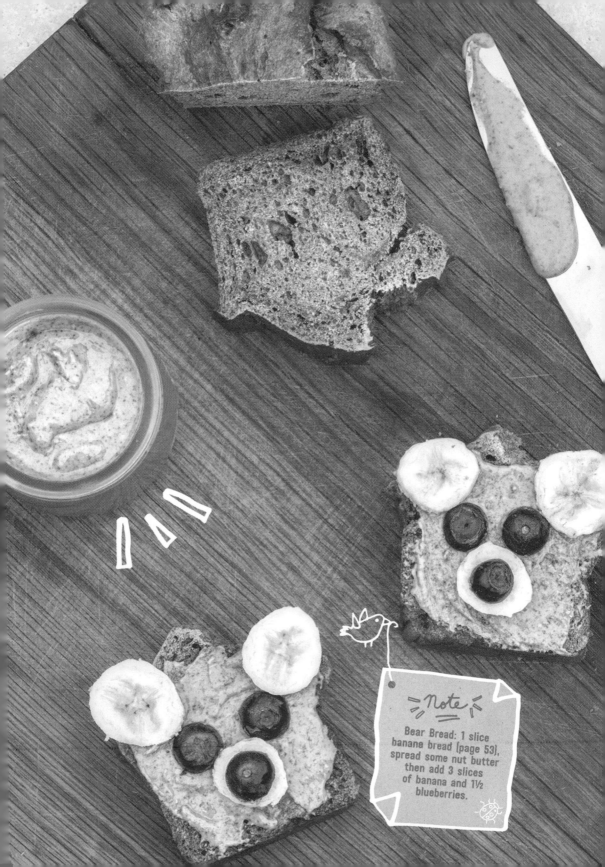

Note

Bear Bread: 1 slice banane bread (page 53), spread some nut butter then add 3 slices of banana and 1½ blueberries.

Nut Butters &
Almondella

Making your own nut butters may seem like a daunting task but it is very easy and requires only the nuts you want to use and a food processor – that's it! For a chocolatey spread, I prefer to use almonds, as they are significantly cheaper than hazelnuts.

Each quantity makes 1 large jar (about 275ml)

Peanut Butter

200g peanuts

Place the peanuts on a baking tray and roast for 10 minutes. Remove from the oven and immediately place into a food processor. Process until they start to release their oils and turn into a smooth butter. This takes about 15 minutes.

Cashew Butter

200g cashew nuts

Place cashews into a food processor and process until they start to release their oils and turn into a smooth butter. This takes about 15 minutes.

Almondella
2 tbsp (40g): 24.2g free sugar
24.2g total in 275g

200g almonds
2 tablespoons maple syrup
1 tablespoon cacao powder

Preheat oven to 180º/350º/gas 4.

Place the almonds on a baking tray and roast for 10 minutes. When finished, immediately place into a food processor and process until they start to release their oils and turn into a smooth butter. This takes about 15 minutes.

When it has become almond butter, add the maple syrup and cacao powder. It will change consistency but keep blending until it becomes smooth and chocolatey.

Serve with Baby Banana Bread (see page 53).

Chia Jam

Chia jam is one of the quickest and most delicious things you can make at home. Forget sugar- and preservative-filled jams and go for this healthier option. It is so zingy and perfect on toast or pancakes for a healthy baby treat.

Makes 1 medium jar (about 185ml)

2 tsp (5g): 3g free sugar
3g total in 185ml

300g summer berries

½ lemon, juice only

2 tablespoons maple syrup

2 tablespoons chia seeds

Add all of the ingredients, except for the chia seeds, to a saucepan and bring to the boil. Turn down to a medium heat and stir often, until the mixture starts to thicken and turns into a syrup. It will take anywhere from 12–15 minutes.

Add the chia seeds to the saucepan and allow to bubble away for a further 5 minutes, stirring well to prevent sticking.

Transfer the jam to a sterilised jar and tap to remove any air pockets. Then seal and store in the fridge.

Serve on pancakes or bread, in yogurt or over porridge.

☆ ☆ ☆

Easy Apple Sauce

This is a staple snack in our house – I always have some around. It's simple to make and so tasty and nutritious.

Makes 1 medium jar (about 185ml)

4 sweet eating apples, washed and cut into small chunks

4 tablespoons water

¼ teaspoon cinnamon

Place all the ingredients in a saucepan and bring to the boil. This only takes a few minutes. Immediately turn the heat down and cover the saucepan with a lid.

Simmer for 10 minutes and then transfer the mixture to a NutriBullet or blender and blend until beautifully smooth.

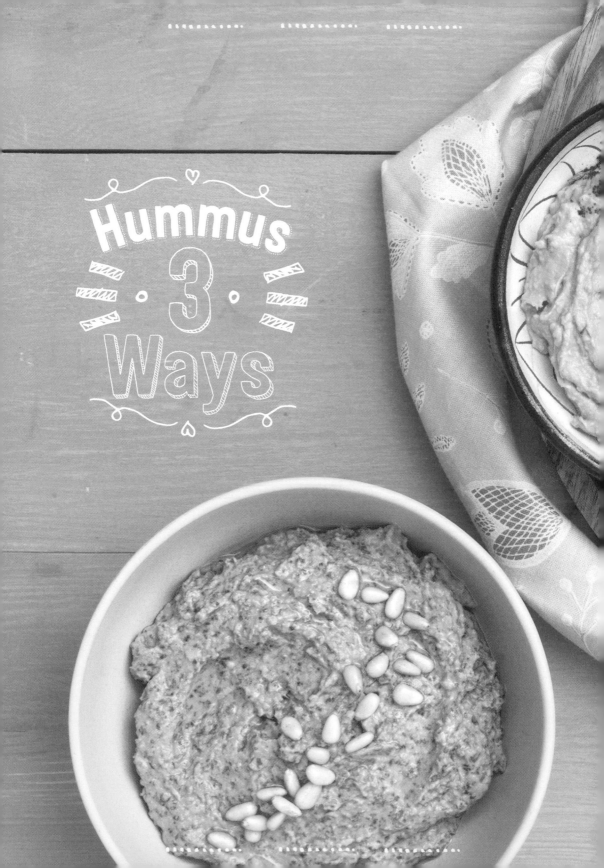

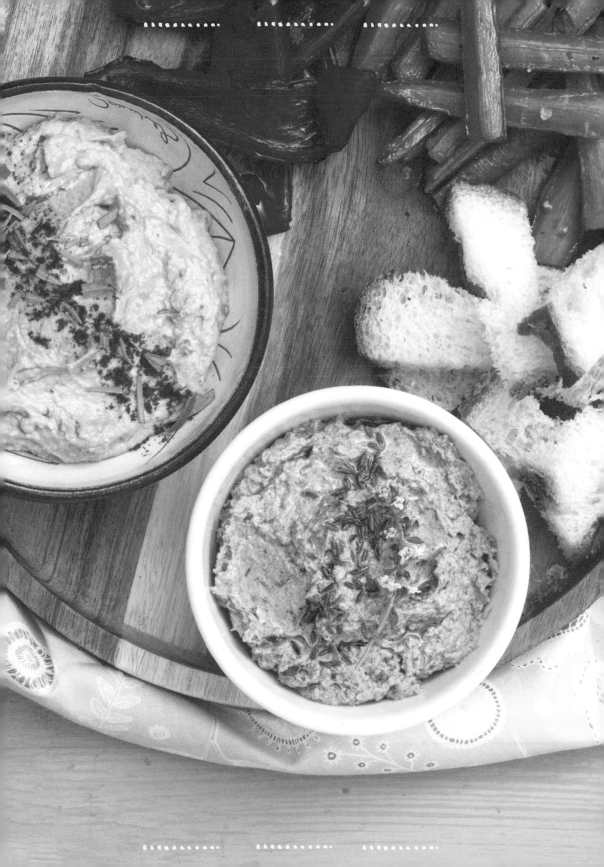

Hummus
3 Ways

Hummus is one of my favourite healthy dips, and when added to a salad and some chicken it can transform a regular meal into a really delicious one. Not only that but hummus is also great as a vegan butter and works well with steamed veggie sticks. Babies love dipping!

Makes 500g

Super Green Hummus

6 cloves garlic, skin on

400g tinned chickpeas

4 tablespoons tahini

4 tablespoons extra virgin olive oil

4 tablespoons water

1 lemon, juice only

60g spinach

40g kale leaves

20g parsley

Preheat oven to 180°C/350°/gas 4.

Place the garlic on a baking tray and bake for 15–20 minutes until soft. Then remove from the oven and pop the cloves out of their skins.

Add all of the ingredients to a food processor and process until the hummus is deliciously creamy.

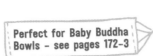

Perfect for Baby Buddha
Bowls – see pages 172–3

Sweet Potato Hummus

6 cloves garlic, skin on

400g tinned chickpeas

4 tablespoons tahini

4 tablespoons extra virgin
olive oil

4 tablespoons water

1 lemon, juice only

400g cooked sweet potato

large sprig rosemary,
leaves picked

Preheat oven to 180°/350°/gas 4.

Place the garlic on a baking tray and bake for 15–20 minutes until soft. Then remove from the oven and pop the cloves out of their skins.

Add all of the ingredients to a food processor and process until the hummus is deliciously creamy.

Curried Aubergine Hummus

8 cloves garlic, skin on

2 aubergines, thinly sliced

400g tinned chickpeas

4 tablespoons tahini

4 tablespoons extra virgin
olive oil

4 tablespoons water

1 lemon, juice only

1 teaspoon ground cumin

1 teaspoon mild curry
powder

½ teaspoon garam masala

Preheat oven to 180°/350°/gas 4.

Place the garlic and aubergine on a baking tray, drizzle with a little olive oil and bake for 15 minutes, until the aubergine is soft and starting to turn dark. Remove from the oven and pop the cloves out of their skins.

Add all of the ingredients to a food processor and process until the hummus is deliciously creamy.

Pesto

3 Ways

Pesto is another one of those recipes that once you make at home you won't ever buy again. Just put everything into a blender, whizz it up until it turns into a deliciously silky sauce and pour over pasta or meat or – one of my favourites – put in a toasted sandwich with mozzarella and cherry tomatoes. Some of these recipes use pumpkin seeds instead of pine nuts, and I also use a good goat's cheese instead of Parmesan, which is too salty for little weaning babies.

Each quantity makes 1 medium jar (about 185ml)

Red Pepper and Goat's Cheese Pesto

2 red peppers, cut into strips

6 cloves garlic, skins on

20g hard goat's cheese, grated

70ml extra virgin olive oil

60g pine nuts

20g basil leaves

Preheat oven to 180°C.

Place the peppers on a baking tray, drizzle with a little olive oil and scatter the cloves of garlic through them. Bake for 25 minutes, until the peppers are soft and cooked.

Remove the garlic cloves from their skins, place all the ingredients into a blender and blend until smooth and silky.

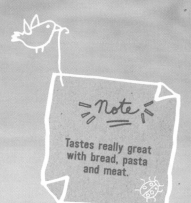

Note

Tastes really great with bread, pasta and meat.

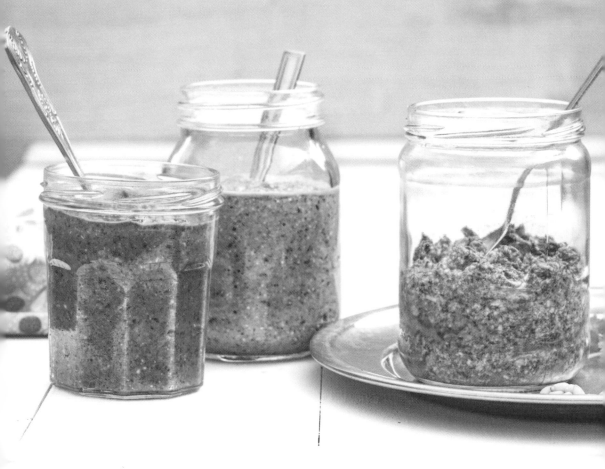

Please turn over

Roasted Tomato and Aubergine Pesto

1 aubergine, cut into 1cm slices

3 plum tomatoes

6 cloves garlic, skins on

20g basil leaves

60g pine nuts

70ml extra virgin olive oil, plus extra for drizzling

¼ teaspoon paprika

Preheat oven to 180°C/350°/gas 4.

Drizzle the aubergine slices with a little olive oil and grill on each side until slightly browned.

Place the tomatoes and garlic on a baking tray and bake for 25 minutes until the garlic is soft and the tomatoes are bursting with juice. Remove the garlic from the skins then place all of the ingredients into a blender and blend until the sauce becomes smooth and silky.

Spinach and Kale Pesto

6 cloves garlic, skins on

40g kale

40g spinach

160ml extra virgin olive oil

small bunch parsley

40g toasted pumpkin seeds

20g hard goat's cheese, grated

Preheat oven to 180°C/350°/gas 4.

Place the garlic onto a baking tray and bake for 25 minutes. Remove the garlic from the skins, then add it and all the other ingredients to a blender. Blend until smooth and silky.

Guacamole

Once you try this guacamole, you will never want the store-bought kind again. It takes less than 5 minutes to prepare – just chop, squeeze and stir. It makes the perfect accompaniment to Huevos Rancheros (see page 49) or Mexican Taquitos (see page 161).

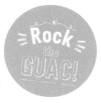

Serves 2 adults and 2 children

1 ripe avocado

small bunch fresh coriander, finely chopped (including stalks)

½ lime, juice only

½ small sweet onion, finely chopped

pinch black pepper

4 cherry tomatoes, finely diced

Mash the avocado in a bowl, add the rest of the ingredients and stir well. Easy and yummy!

Black Bean Dip

This takes 5 minutes to cook and tastes so much better than any store-bought dip. It is so nutritious and goes beautifully with anything Mexican. It also works really well as a spread for holding veggies in a baby wrap.

Serves 2 adults and 2 children

1 small onion, chopped

2 cloves garlic, crushed

400g tinned unsalted black beans

3 tablespoons olive oil, plus extra for frying

Heat a drizzle of olive oil in a saucepan over a medium heat and gently fry the onion until sweet and sticky.

Add the garlic and beans and fry for a further 2–3 minutes until cooked but not brown.

Transfer the entire mixture, along with the 3 tablespoons of olive oil, to a blender and blend until smooth. Serve straight away.

Spinach & Garlic
Creamy Dip

If one thing reminds me of Christmas, it's this dip. My mother used to lace it with raw garlic, but this isn't the best for little babies' tummies. Instead I opt for a softer-tasting dip by using roasted garlic along with creamy yogurt and fresh spinach and just a hint of spice. It is so delicious and a great spread for sandwiches – it's definitely not just for Christmas!

Makes 1 medium jar (about 185ml)

200g natural yogurt

2 heaped tablespoons soft goat's cheese

sprinkle black pepper

½ teaspoon Dijon mustard

2 tablespoons parsley, finely chopped

4 cloves roasted garlic, crushed

60g fresh spinach, finely chopped

Place all of the ingredients in a bowl and mix well until the cheese has broken up and it becomes a thick sauce.

Refined-Sugar-Free
Baby Ketchup

When my mam gave me a huge box of her home-grown tomatoes, I felt they were calling me to turn them into something wonderful. I had noticed my older kids' addiction to store-bought ketchup and I was determined to make a healthier alternative that would be more nourishing and wouldn't contain any of the sugar and processed ingredients ketchup normally does. This is a sauce you really won't mind your little ones dipping a chip into.

Makes 1 large jar (about 275ml)

60ml: 36.3g free sugar
36.3g total in 275ml

400g tinned or fresh tomatoes, peeled

6 tablespoons unsalted tomato purée

170ml apple cider vinegar

1 clove garlic

1 teaspoon onion powder

½ teaspoon cinnamon

½ teaspoon ground cloves

60ml maple syrup

Place all of the ingredients in a blender and blend until smooth.

Pour into a saucepan and bring to the boil. Reduce the heat to its lowest setting and simmer without covering. Let the sauce bubble away for an hour, making sure to stir every few minutes. Once the sauce has fully thickened, take it off the heat and leave to cool.

Store in the fridge in a sealed, sterilised jar for up to a month.

Cajun Sauce

This is our go-to sauce for burgers and it goes great with sweet potato fries as well as roasted chicken strips. It's all kinds of yum and so healthy!

Serves 2 adults and 2 children

120ml natural yogurt
1 teaspoon onion powder
1 teaspoon garlic powder
1 teaspoon ground nutmeg
1 teaspoon paprika
¼ teaspoon chilli powder
(optional)

Place all of the ingredients in a bowl and stir really well until the sauce turns pink and the spices are mixed through.

Dollop over burgers and serve.

Toddler-Friendly Asian Dip

This gorgeous dipping sauce is perfect for toddlers for dipping Baby Sushi (see page 178) or Rice-Paper Rolls (see page 176).

Serves 2 adults and 2 children

2 tablespoons peanut butter
2 tablespoons tahini
½ lemon, juice only
2 teaspoons low-sodium soy sauce
1 tablespoon olive oil

Mix everything in a bowl until smooth and creamy and then serve.

Chicken Stock

Homemade stock is so nutritious and has none of the additives used in commercial stocks. It's economical to make and I always have some in the freezer, ready to go!

Makes about 1 litre

1 cooked chicken carcass

2 onions, peeled and roughly chopped

2 carrots, peeled and roughly chopped

2 sticks celery, roughly chopped

large handful kale leaves, roughly chopped

2 bay leaves

12 black peppercorns

Place the chicken carcass into a large pot. Add the rest of the ingredients and enough cold water to just cover the chicken.

Bring to the boil and then cover with a lid and reduce the heat. Simmer for 2 hours. Allow to fully cool then place a sieve over a large bowl and strain the mixture in. Discard the bones and vegetables.

Portion the stock into a silicone muffin tin and freeze. Remove the portions from the silicone tin and place into freezer bags until ready to use.

Yummy
Treats

for Little Hands

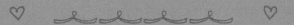

Refined-sugar-free, simple to make

treats and snacks

that are not only natural but also super tasty.
These yummy baby-friendly, family treats will
have everyone eating healthier in no time.

From homemade teething pops to delicious
chocolate and muffins there is a recipe for
every occasion and even a few that sneak
•••• more veggies into little tummies. ••••

Yummy Scrummy
in My Tummy Gummies

These little gummies are made using only fresh fruit, vanilla and gelatine. They are softer than the regular shop-bought kinds and contain only sugar from the fruit, making them the healthiest jelly you could possibly give your baby.

Each recipe makes about 100 gummies

Mango Gummies

1 medium ready-to-eat mango, peeled and stone removed

60ml lemon juice, freshly squeezed

2 teaspoons vanilla extract

3 tablespoons grass-fed gelatine

Blackberry Gummies

250g blackberries

60ml lemon juice, freshly squeezed

2 teaspoons vanilla extract

3 tablespoons grass-fed gelatine

Place your chosen fruit in a blender with the lemon juice and vanilla extract. Blend until completely smooth and silky. The mixture should measure roughly 250ml – if it measures more, leave the excess aside. If using blackberries, sieve the mixture to remove the seeds.

Pour the fruit mixture into a saucepan and heat until it starts to bubble. It is important not to boil it, as this will destroy the vitamin C. Stir thoroughly to make sure the entire mixture is hot and then remove from the heat.

Sprinkle over the gelatine and whisk slowly until it is completely dissolved.

Pour into sweet moulds and then place in the refrigerator until completely set. Store in the fridge in an airtight jar – they will last for 4 days (if you hide them from the kids).

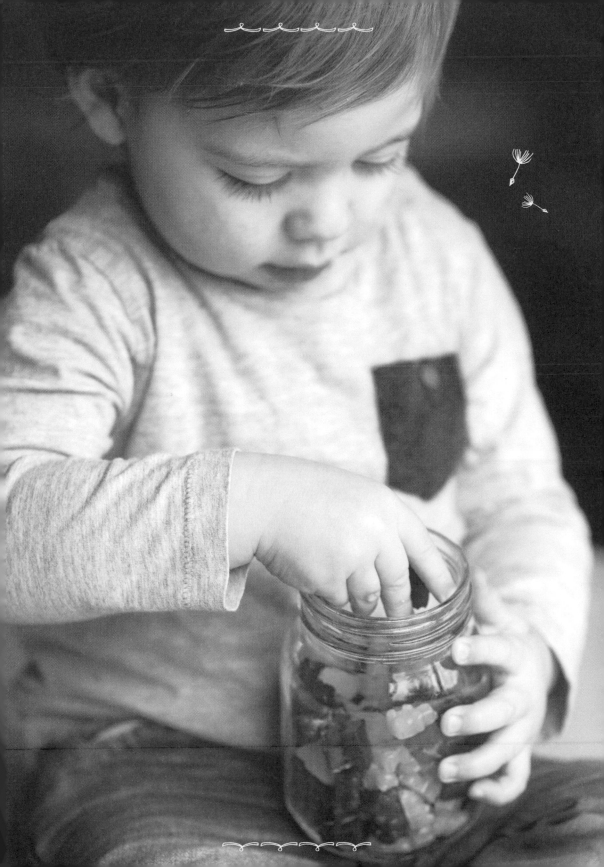

Fruit & Veggie
Roll-Ups

These are ideal treats for little ones. There's no added sugar or crazy preservatives and kids of all ages love them. They're made using not only fruit but also hidden veggies, making them really nutritious. There is nothing better than hearing your kids ask for another green one (yes, of course you can have another kale, beetroot and berry sweet!).

Each recipe makes about 12

Mango and Passion Fruit
200g mango flesh, chopped

2 passion fruit, flesh only

Beetroot, Kale, Blueberry and Grape
100g raw beetroot, washed, peeled and roughly chopped

40g kale leaves

100g grapes

80g blueberries

Kiwi, Spinach and Lime
300g kiwi, peeled

40g spinach leaves

1 ripe pear, peeled, cored and roughly chopped

1 lime, juice only

Apple and Cinnamon
4 sweet eating apples, peeled, cored and roughly chopped

¼ teaspoon cinnamon

Preheat oven to its lowest setting (mine goes down to 80°C).

Choose the roll-up you are going to make, add all of the ingredients to a blender and blend until really smooth, without any lumps whatsoever. Have a little taste and make sure you are happy with the sweetness. You can always add a teaspoon of maple syrup if it isn't sweet enough.

Line a baking tray with parchment paper, pour the fruit/vegetable sauce in and spread evenly. It shouldn't be too thick – just about ½ centimetre deep.

Place the tray in the oven and leave it for about 6 hours. It should dry out completely and have no wet patches. After 3 hours, check it every hour until it is totally dry. Cooking time will vary depending on the thickness of the fruit and oven temperature.

When it is totally dry, remove from the oven and allow to cool fully. Then cut the roll-ups into long strips and peel off the parchment paper.

Store in an airtight container and use within 1 week.

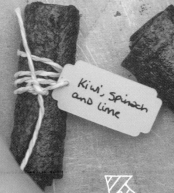

Beetroot, Kale,
Blueberries &
Grape :)

Apple &
Cinnamon

Mango &
Passion Fruit :)

Kiwi, Spinach
and Lime

yum...

Sweet Potato
Truffles

This is one of my all-time favourite creations. It may sound odd to make sweets from sweet potato but, seriously, they are amazing! Sweet and orangey and totally fabulous, they are the ultimate healthy treat for your family.

Makes 42 truffles

1 tbsp (20g): 12.1g free sugar
(42 servings) 0.28g each

For the filling

6 Medjool dates, pitted and chopped

6 tablespoons coconut oil

1 teaspoon orange-blossom water or vanilla extract

½ orange, zest and juice

200g roast sweet potato, puréed

4 tablespoons coconut flour

For the chocolate coating

100g cacao butter

1 teaspoon orange-blossom water or vanilla extract

1 tablespoon maple syrup

1½ tablespoons cacao powder

3 tablespoons tahini

2 tablespoons cashew butter

Preheat oven to 180°C/350°F/gas 4.

Place the dates, coconut oil, orange-blossom water, zest and juice in a saucepan and bring to the boil.

Reduce the heat to medium and keep stirring until the dates break down and the mixture starts to look like a thick caramel. The oil will separate but that's OK.

Pour the mixture into a bowl and add the puréed sweet potato and coconut flour and stir until it becomes nice and thick.

Roll the mixture into 42 little balls and put a cocktail stick into each one to make dunking into the chocolate easier – it keeps them clean and smudge free. Place into the fridge again until you're ready to dunk.

Place the cacao butter, orange-blossom water and maple syrup in a bowl over a saucepan a quarter full of simmering water. Make sure the water doesn't touch the bowl.

When the cacao butter has melted, take off the heat and add the cacao powder, tahini and cashew butter and stir well until totally soft and chocolatey. Leave the chocolate in the fridge for 5 minutes to allow it to thicken slightly, as it will coat the truffles better.

Remove the truffles from the fridge and dunk each one until completely covered and then place on parchment paper to set.

Eat! Eat! Eat!

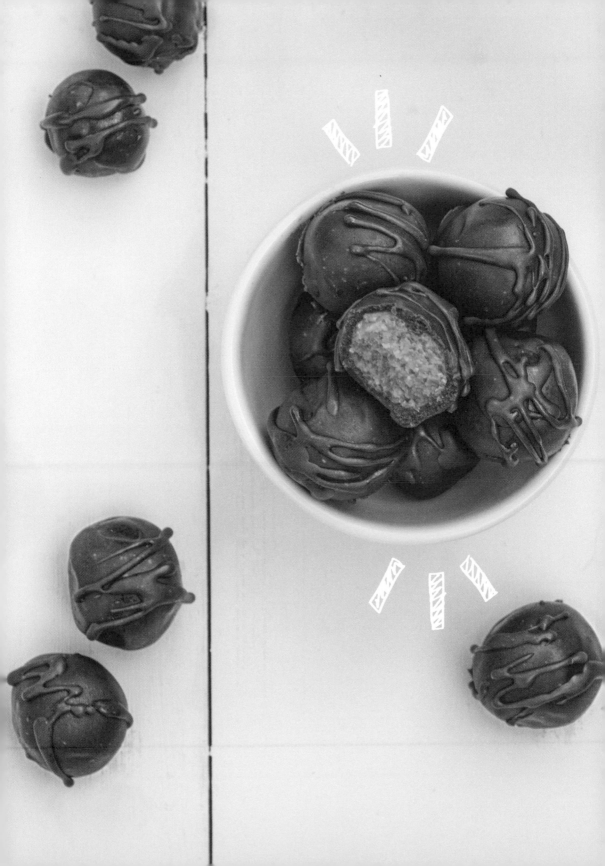

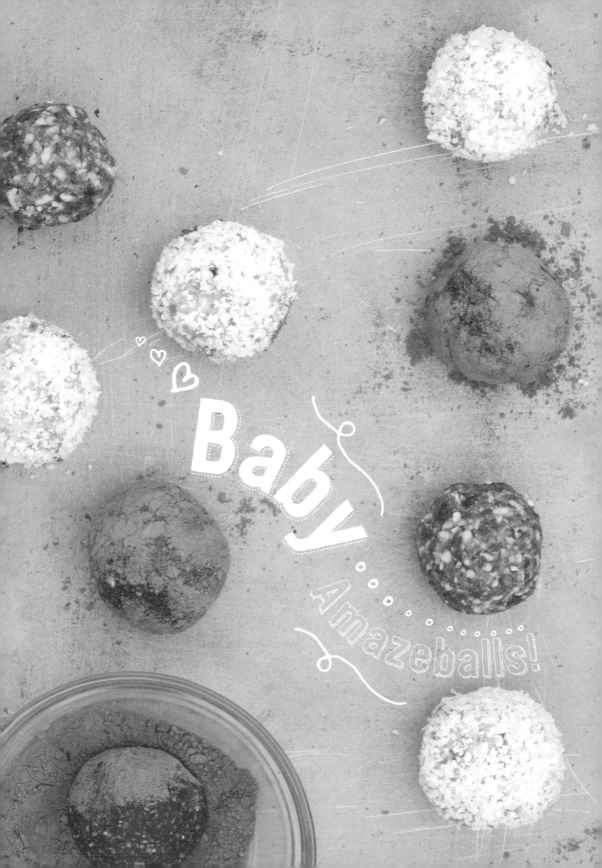

Baby ♡ ♡ ♡ Amazeballs!

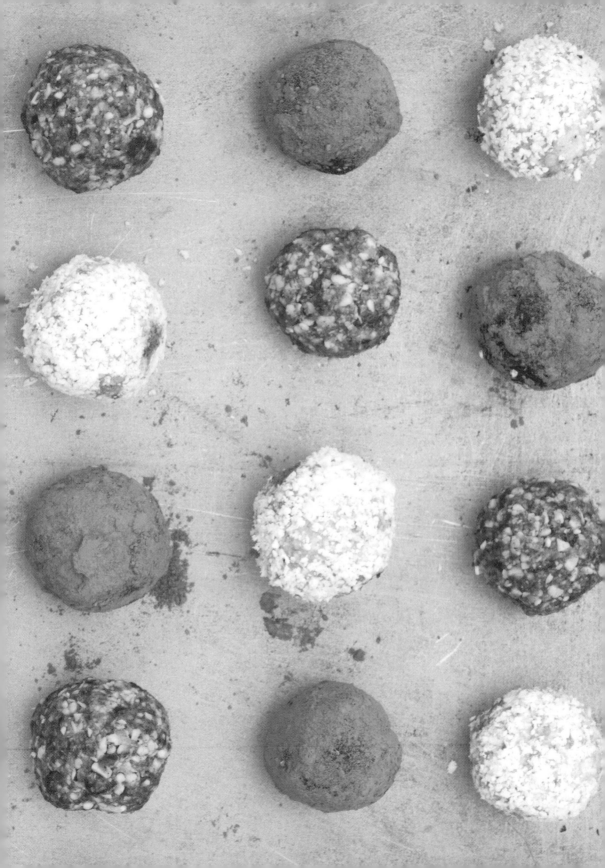

Baby
Amazeballs!

I am known among my friends as the woman who makes the baby amazeballs – I kid you not. These are our go-to weekend treat – small, delicious, sweet balls of yumminess. Below are three of our favourites. They require no baking, only five minutes of mixing, and anyone can make them. I have also included a nut-and-date-free option.

Each recipe makes 12 Amazeballs

Lemon Sorbet Amazeballs:
2 tbsp (40g) : 24.2g free sugar
(12 servings) 2g each

Gingerbread Amazeballs

8 Medjool dates, pitted

140g almonds

50g oats

1 teaspoon ground ginger

½ teaspoon ground allspice (or cinnamon)

5 tablespoons melted coconut oil

Lemon Sorbet Amazeballs (nut free)

100g sunflower seeds

1 lemon, zest and juice

2 tablespoons maple syrup

80g oats

80g coconut

5 tablespoons melted coconut oil

½ teaspoon turmeric

Chocolate Orange Amazeballs

160g almonds

8 Medjool dates, pitted

50g oats

2 tablespoons cacao powder

1 orange, zest of whole orange and juice of ½

Choose the recipe you are going to make, place all the ingredients into a food processor and process until really fine and coming together like a dough. If it is a little dry, add some water, just one tablespoon at a time.

Turn the mixture out onto a board, form into a ball and divide into 12 equal parts (I use a knife for this). Using your hands, roll each piece into a ball and place them on a small plate.

When you are finished, put the amazeballs into the fridge for a couple of hours to set. Store in the fridge in an airtight container for 5–7 days.

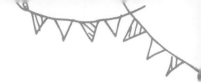

Yummy
Almond Milk

One of my favourite things from one of the people I admire most – this almond milk recipe comes from the fabulous Susan Jane White.

Makes 700–900ml

140g raw almonds
700ml filtered water
2 Medjool dates, pitted
½ teaspoon vanilla extract
1 nut-milk bag

Place the almonds in a large bowl. Cover with cold filtered water and soak overnight or for 10–12 hours.

Rinse and drain, then place in a blender with the 700ml filtered water, dates and vanilla. Blend furiously for 15 seconds.

Wash your hands thoroughly before the next step to avoid spoiling the milk. Pour it into a nut-milk bag set inside a large bowl. Secure the top of the bag and use your fingers to squeeze all the liquid from the pulp.

Discard the dry pulp and pour the creamy milk into a scrupulously clean bottle with a screw-top lid. Store in the fridge and drink within three days.

Frozen Yogurt
Buttons

Essentially just frozen yogurt and fruit in the shape of little buttons, these little treats are a healthy alternative to sugary sweets and are brilliant for little teething gums.

Makes about 30

1 ripe banana

1 teaspoon vanilla extract

10 strawberries, hulled

125ml Greek yogurt

Add the banana, vanilla and strawberries to a blender and blend until you have a smooth purée.

Pour into a bowl, add the yogurt and mix well. (Do not blend the yogurt as it will make the mixture too runny.)

Cover a plate with cling film. Pour the mixture into a piping bag and pipe little drops of the yogurt mixture onto the cling film.

Put the plate into the freezer and freeze until drops are solid. Peel them off the cling film and keep in a covered container in the freezer.

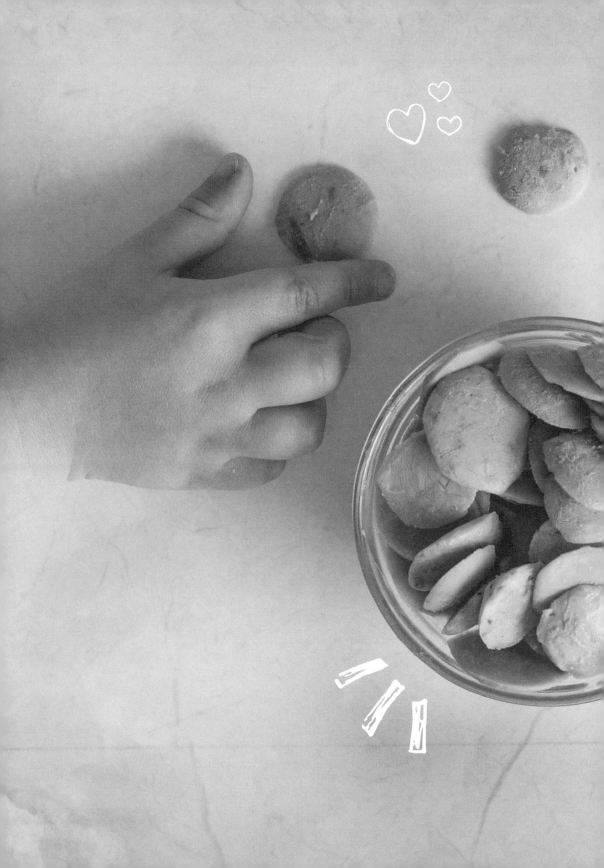

Coconut Milk
Ice-Cream Sambos

These ice-cream sandwiches are baby-friendly treats filled with vitamins, minerals and healthy sugars (from the sweetness of ripe bananas). They're perfect for a hot summer's day and cool sore, teething gums without filling your baby full of refined sugars.

Makes 12 sandwiches

100ml: 60.7g free sugar
(12 servings) 5g each

400ml full-fat tinned coconut milk, unshaken and refrigerated for 2 hours

2 bananas, sliced and frozen

2 teaspoons vanilla extract

100g oat flour

150g buckwheat flour

1 teaspoon baking powder

1 teaspoon vanilla

1 tablespoon linseeds

100ml maple syrup

120g coconut oil, melted

3 tablespoons cacao powder

80g almond/peanut butter

To make the ice-cream, carefully open the can of coconut milk and scoop the cream that's formed above the milk into a bowl – reserve the milk and the can for later.

Gently whisk the coconut cream until peaks start to form.

To a blender, add the frozen bananas, vanilla and half the reserved coconut milk, and blend until the mixture is soft and silky. Then fold the banana mixture into the whipped coconut cream.

Pour the mixture into the empty coconut-milk can, cover with cling film and place in the freezer until frozen (2–4 hours).

Meanwhile, add the flours and baking powder to a large bowl, make a well in the centre and add the remaining ingredients. Using a wooden spoon, mix well until it forms a dough.

Turn onto a floured surface and roll out to 1cm thick. Cut out 12 circles, roughly 7cm in diameter.

Place onto a tray lined with parchment paper and bake for 12 minutes. Leave to cool fully.

To assemble the ice-cream sambos, take the tin out of the freezer. Remove the cling film and run the sides of the tin under a warm tap for just a few seconds – the ice-cream should slide out easily.

Cut the ice-cream into 1.5cm slices and place a biscuit either side. Wrap individually in cling film and store in the freezer.

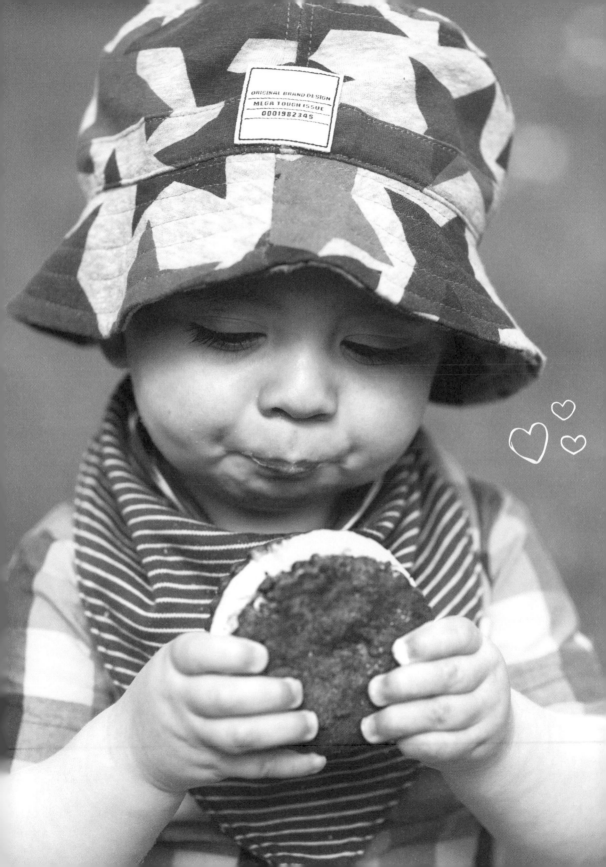

Peach & Lavender
Coconut Milk Ice-Cream

Since I started writing my cookbook, I have been offering food over the garden fence to our lovely neighbours, getting them to taste test to make sure it's not just my family who like the recipes. When they saw me in our flower bed picking lavender buds they joked if I was using them for food. Imagine their surprise when over the fence, later that day, came the most delicious dairy-free, sugar-free lavender ice-cream. The taste of lavender is quite mild but, I promise, totally amazing and worth it!

Makes 500ml

3 ripe peaches, cut in half and stoned

1 teaspoon vanilla extract

5g lavender buds

800ml full-fat tinned coconut milk, unshaken and refrigerated for 2 hours

Preheat oven to 180°C/350°F/gas 4.

Place peach halves skin-side down on a baking tray. Bake for 25 minutes until they are soft. This makes them even sweeter and yummier!

When they are cooked, put the peaches into a blender along with the vanilla and lavender. Blend until smooth and silky. Have a taste and make sure it is sweet enough. If not, add a little maple syrup. My peaches were really ripe so they didn't need anything extra. Leave aside to fully cool.

Carefully open the cans of coconut milk and scoop out the cream that's formed above the milk into a bowl. Gently whisk the coconut cream until firm peaks start to form.

Fold the peach mixture into the coconut cream, ensuring that it is totally combined. Then pour into a tin lined with parchment paper, cover tightly with cling-film and freeze for at least 4 hours until firm.

To serve, take the ice-cream out of the freezer and allow to thaw slightly. Scoop out baby-sized portions and serve.

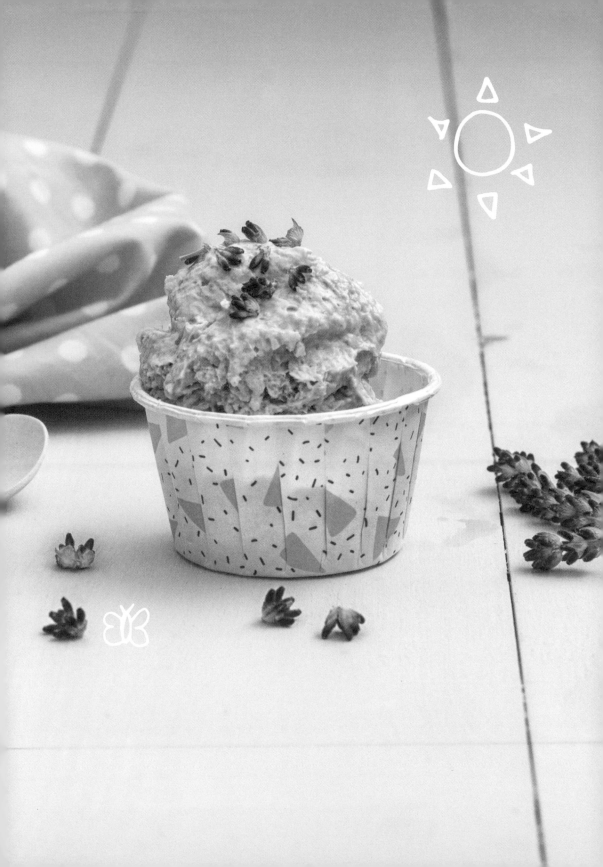

Mango Ice-Cream

On a summer's day, there is nothing nicer than ice-cream. Cooling and deliciously creamy, it's usually packed with crazy amounts of sugar so I wanted to create a relatively healthy option but made in the same way as traditional ice-cream. The knack to great ice-cream, I've learned, is to make sure the custard is as cold as possible before adding to your ice-cream maker.

Makes 1 litre

3 tbsp (60g): 36.3g free sugar
36.3g total in 1 litre

500ml double cream

250ml whole milk

4 egg yolks

3 tablespoons maple syrup

1 tablespoon vanilla extract

1 ripe mango, skinned and stone removed

½ teaspoon turmeric

Pour the cream and milk into a saucepan and heat gently over a medium heat. Place the egg yolks into a bowl and beat with the maple syrup and vanilla until smooth and creamy.

To ensure the egg yolks don't curdle, do not add them to the milk and cream. Instead, remove about 250ml of the warm milk mixture and whisk into the egg yolks, then pour this into the saucepan of warm milk, whisking as you do.

Heat gently, stirring all the time. The mixture will start to thicken, which will take about 15 minutes. It should cling to the back of a metal spoon and have the consistency of custard.

Pour into a bowl, immediately cover with cling-film and leave in the fridge for about 4 hours to get really cold.

Meanwhile, in a blender, purée the mango with the turmeric. When the custard is fully cooled add half the purée to the mixture and stir well.

Pour the mixture into an ice-cream machine and churn as per the instructions until it is thick. Pour into a tin lined with parchment paper.

Spoon blobs of the remaining mango mixture over the ice-cream and draw a butter knife through to swirl them throughout.

Cover with cling film and freeze until hard.

To serve, take the ice-cream out of the freezer to thaw slightly, making it easier to scoop out servings.

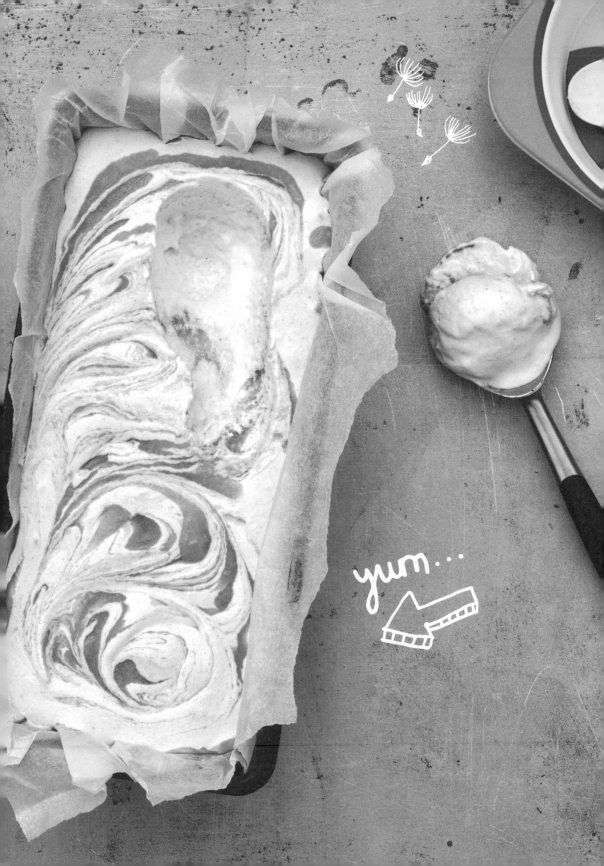

yum...

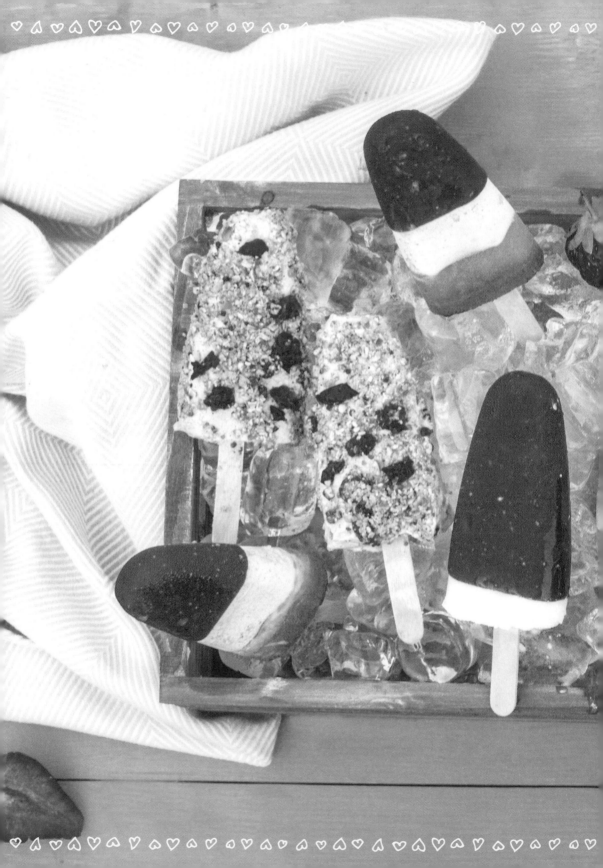

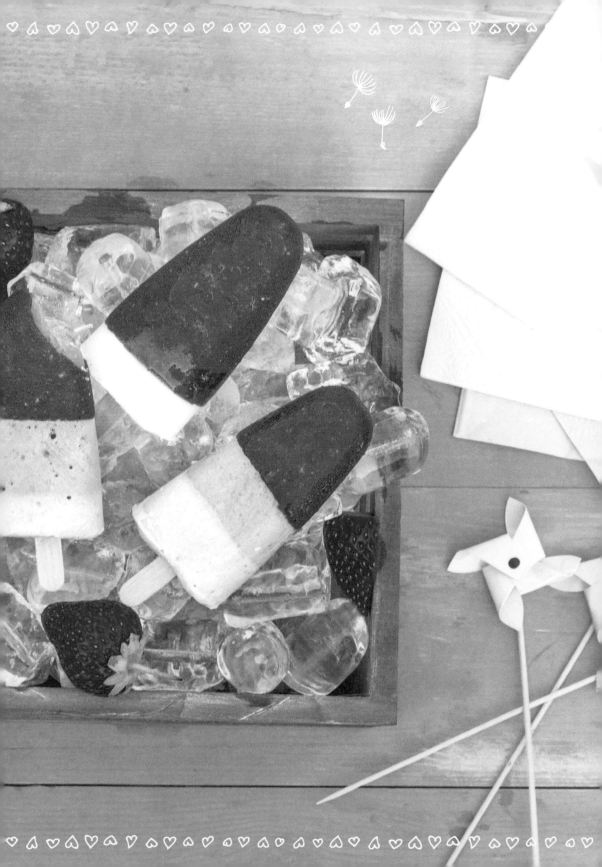

Ireland's Favourite
Ice-Pops made in a healthier way

In Ireland, sunny days and ice-pops just go hand in hand. These recipes are my take on the favourite ice-pops we've enjoyed in this country over the years – without all the sugar and flavourings. These are naturally healthy and delicious treats you won't mind reaching into the freezer for.

Each recipe makes 12 ice-pops

Loop the Loop (Dairy Free)

2 tbsp (40g): 24.2g free sugar
50g Baby Chocolate: 4.84g
(12 servings) 2.42g each

Lemon sorbet layer

400ml full-fat tinned coconut milk

½ teaspoon turmeric

1 tablespoon maple syrup

1 lemon, zest and juice

Lime ice-pop layer

1 lime, zest and juice

10 spinach leaves

1 tablespoon maple syrup

80ml water

Chocolate layer

50g Baby Chocolate (see page 236)

To make the lemon sorbet, place the coconut milk into the fridge overnight. The next morning, carefully open the tin, making sure not to shake it, then scoop out the coconut cream from the top (the lovely thick part).

Whisk until light and fluffy, and then whisk in the turmeric, maple syrup, lemon zest and juice. Half fill the moulds with the mixture then put an ice-pop stick in each and freeze.

To make the lime ice-pop, add all of the ingredients to a blender and blend until the spinach leaves have completely broken up and the liquid is psychedelic green. Fill the remaining half of the moulds up and then freeze until solid.

For the chocolate layer, melt the chocolate in a bowl over a saucepan a quarter full of simmering water. Make sure the water doesn't touch the bowl. Remove from the heat and pour the chocolate into a glass. This makes it easier to dip. Put the chocolate in the fridge or freezer for about 5 minutes until it has cooled but not set.

Remove the ice-pops from the freezer and take them out of the moulds. Dip the ice-pops halfway into the chocolate. Because the pops are frozen the chocolate should harden straight away. Store in the freezer until ready to serve.

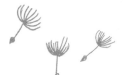

Wibbly Wobbly Wonder

2 tbsp (40g): 24.2g free sugar
50g Baby Chocolate: 4.84g
(12 servings) 2.42g each

Lemon jelly

1 tablespoon grass-fed gelatine

4 tablespoons water

100g mango flesh

1 lemon, juice only

120ml water

2 tablespoons maple syrup

½ teaspoon turmeric

Strawberry ice-cream

150ml milk

1 banana

80g fresh strawberries, hulled

Banana ice-cream

150ml milk

2 bananas

50g Baby Chocolate (see page 236)

To make the lemon jelly, add the gelatine to the 4 tablespoons of water, stir quickly and leave aside for a few minutes to thicken up completely.

Add all of the remaining ingredients to a blender and blend until smooth and fully combined. Pour the mixture into a saucepan. Bring to the boil, then remove from the heat and stir in the gelatine until it has fully dissolved.

Pour the mixture into the ice-pop moulds, filling up only a quarter of the way. Put an ice-pop stick in each and freeze until solid. (I used cling-film over the moulds to hold the sticks in place.)

Next, to make the strawberry ice-cream, add the milk, banana and strawberries to a blender and blend until smooth and creamy. Pour into the ice-cream moulds, filling up to about three-quarters full. Then place into the freezer again and freeze until solid.

For the banana ice-cream, add the milk and banana to a blender and blend until smooth and creamy. Pour into the moulds, filling to the top, then freeze until solid.

Melt the chocolate in a bowl over a saucepan a quarter full of simmering water. Make sure the water doesn't touch the bowl. Remove from the heat and pour the chocolate into a glass. This makes it easier to dip. Put the chocolate in the fridge or freezer for about 5 minutes until it is cooled but not set.

Remove the ice-pops from the freezer and take them out of the moulds. Dip the ice-pops into the chocolate, just covering the jelly layer. Because the pops are frozen, the chocolate should harden straight away. Store in the freezer until ready to serve.

Brunch

250ml milk

1 banana

120g fresh strawberries, hulled

6 tablespoons Baby Fine Granola (see page 42)

2 tablespoons goji berries

6 tbsp Baby Fine Granola: 9g free sugar (12 servings) 0.75g each

Add the milk, banana and strawberries to a blender and blend until smooth and creamy. Pour into ice-cream moulds then put an ice-pop stick in the centre of each and freeze.

Meanwhile, place the granola in a pestle and mortar along with the goji berries and crush until they resemble breadcrumbs.

When the pops are fully frozen, take them out of the freezer and remove from the moulds. Allow them to thaw very slightly and then dip each one into the granola mixture until fully coated. Store in the freezer until ready to serve.

Choc Ice (Dairy Free)

800ml full-fat tinned coconut milk

2 tablespoons maple syrup

1 tablespoon vanilla extract

50g Baby Chocolate (see page 236)

2 tbsp (40g): 24.2g free sugar
50g Baby Chocolate: 4.84g
(12 servings) 2.42g each

Place the tins of coconut milk into the fridge overnight. The next morning, carefully open them, making sure not to shake, and scoop out the coconut cream from the top (the lovely thick part). Add to a bowl along with the maple syrup and vanilla.

Whisk until light and fluffy and spoon into ice-pop moulds. Tap them on the counter to remove any bubbles and, if needed, add more of the cream mixture. Pop a stick into each one and freeze until solid (about 4 hours).

Melt the chocolate in a bowl over a saucepan a quarter full of simmering water. Make sure the water doesn't touch the bowl. Remove from the heat and pour the chocolate into a glass. This makes it easier to dip. Put the chocolate in the fridge or freezer for about 5 minutes until it is cooled but not set.

Remove the ice-pops from the freezer and take them out of the moulds. Dip the ice-pops in almost fully, leaving just a little white showing at the end. Because the pops are frozen, the chocolate should harden straight away. Store in the freezer until ready to serve.

Frozen Banana Pops

Banana pops are a delicious way to soothe your baby's teething gums and they are very healthy too. You can use whatever toppings you like but our favourites are goji berries, coconut, nuts or – a tip I learned from Susan Jane White – raspberry-leaf herbal tea. Much cheaper than using freeze-dried raspberries and deliciously zingy.

Makes 8 pops

125g Baby Chocolate: 12.1g free sugar (8 servings) 1.5g each

4 bananas

8 ice-pop sticks

125g Baby Chocolate (see page 236)

To decorate

ground goji berries, desiccated coconut, ground hazelnuts or ground pure raspberry-leaf herbal tea

Cut each banana in half and push an ice-pop stick into the flat end of each one. Lay them on a plate or tray, place in the freezer and freeze until hard (about 4 hours).

When the bananas are ready, melt the chocolate in a bowl over a saucepan a quarter full of simmering water. Make sure the water doesn't touch the bowl.

Dip each of the banana sticks halfway into the melted chocolate and sprinkle over the topping of your choice. Place on a tray lined with baking parchment and store in the freezer until ready to eat.

delicious...

Avocado Choc Pops

The perfect way to hide avocados for little ones, like mine, who aren't fond of them. No, my baby does not like everything, but I still try and sneak avocados into his diet whatever way I can. These deliciously creamy, chocolatey pops have the added bonus of being packed full of vitamins, minerals and healthy fats. Ice-pops that are good for you and your little one – who would have thought it?

Makes 6 pops

1 ripe avocado

2 teaspoons vanilla extract

200ml full-fat tinned coconut milk

1 tablespoon cacao powder

4 Medjool dates, pitted

Baby Fine Granola, to decorate (see page 42)

Blend all of the ingredients except the granola in a high-speed blender until smooth and creamy, then divide into your ice-pop moulds.

Freeze for at least 4 hours until hard.

To decorate, take each pop out of its mould. Dampen the top with water and dip into the granola before serving.

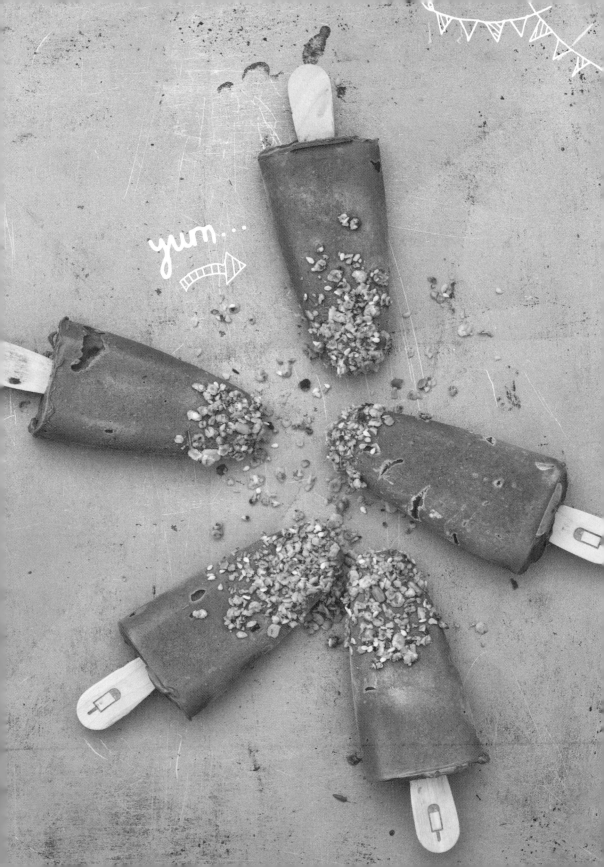

Chocolate
Watermelon Pops

What is there not to like about delicious watermelon covered in healthy chocolate and topped with hazelnuts (if you choose to use them)? These are the perfect way to cool down on a summer's day, and when the kids ask for more you won't mind giving in.

Makes 12 pops

125g Baby Chocolate: 12.1g free sugar (12 servings) 1g each

1 medium-sized watermelon

12 ice-pop sticks

125g Baby Chocolate (see page 236)

ground hazelnuts, to decorate

Cut the watermelon into 1-inch-thick slices then cut the slices into wedges. Push the ice-pop sticks into the skin side of the watermelon.

Melt the chocolate in a bowl over a saucepan a quarter full of simmering water. Make sure the water doesn't touch the bowl. Dip the watermelon halfway into the chocolate and sprinkle over the hazelnuts. Place on a plate lined with baking parchment and refrigerate for at least an hour until the chocolate is set.

Serve straight from the fridge.

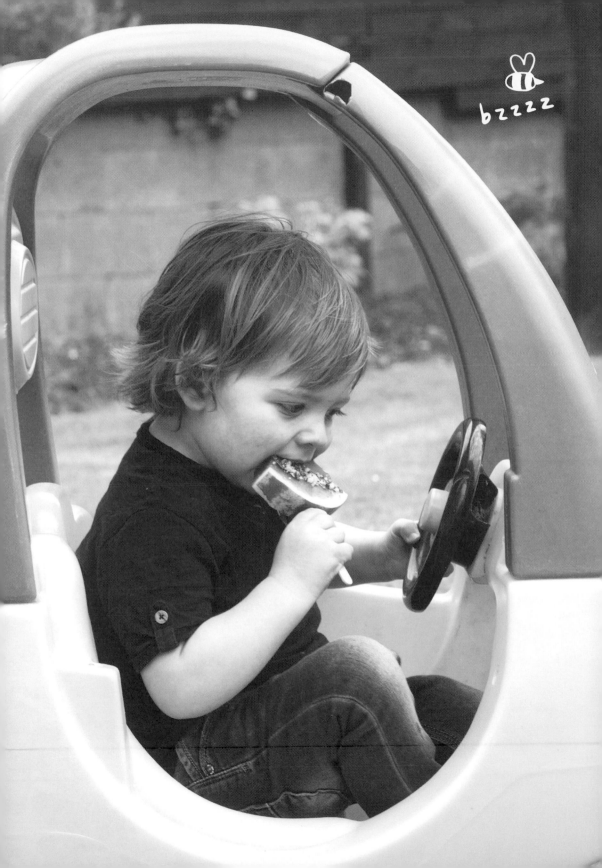

bzzzz

Baby Chocolate

This is the most-read recipe on my Baby-Led Feeding website. It is a little different to the normal dark, natural chocolate you can buy in the store. I use tahini and cashew butter to transform the chocolate into a rich, creamy sauce which sets into the most amazing chocolate you will ever taste.

Makes 250g

2 tbsp (40g): 24.2g free sugar
24.2g total in 250g

100g cacao butter

2 tablespoons maple syrup

1 teaspoon vanilla extract

1 tablespoon cacao powder

3 tablespoons cashew butter (or other smooth nut butter)

2 tablespoons tahini

Bring a saucepan of water, roughly a quarter full, to a boil and then reduce to a simmer. Add the cacao butter to a glass bowl and place over the water to melt, making sure no water gets into the butter and that the water doesn't touch the bottom of the bowl.

Remove from the heat and whisk in the maple syrup, vanilla, cacao powder, cashew butter and tahini until the mixture is completely smooth and creamy.

Pour the mixture into sweet moulds or, alternatively, line a tray with cling film and pour the mixture in.

Place in the fridge for about 2 hours to set or, if you are like me and can't wait, stick it in the freezer for 20 minutes. Store in the fridge in an airtight container for up to a week.

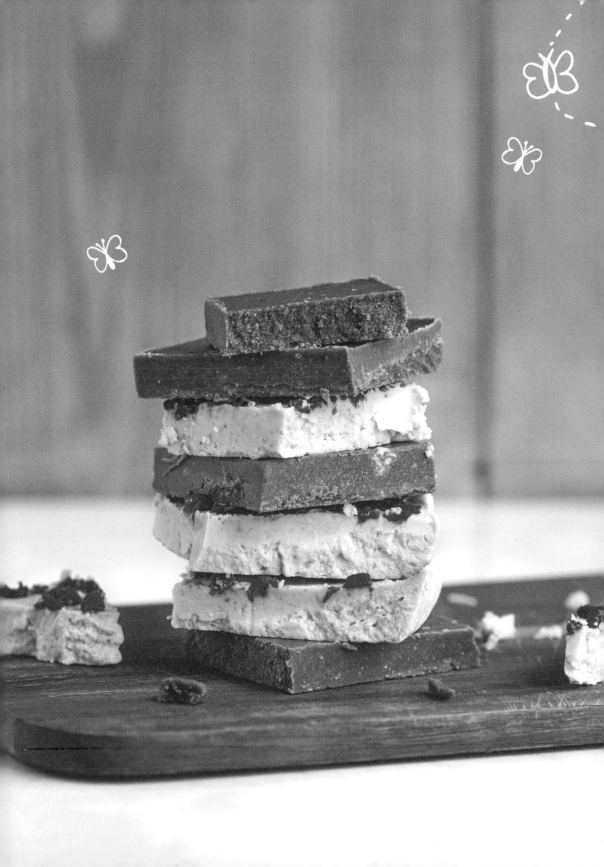

White Chocolate

This white chocolate is totally satisfying and will melt in your little one's mouth just like the shop-bought kind. The difference, though, is that this chocolate is completely refined-sugar free and full of healthy ingredients. The only problem in our house is keeping it away from Daddy!

Makes 250g

2 tbsp (40g): 24.2g free sugar
24.2g total in 250g

100g cacao butter

120g tahini

1 teaspoon vanilla extract

2 tablespoons maple syrup

1 tablespoon goji berries, finely chopped (optional)

Bring a saucepan of water, roughly a quarter full, to a boil and then reduce to a simmer.

Add the cacao butter to a glass bowl and place over the water to melt, making sure no water gets into the butter. It is important to remove the bowl from the heat altogether once the butter has melted, as overheating will destroy the good properties of the butter.

Whisk in the tahini, vanilla and maple syrup until the mixture is completely smooth and creamy.

Pour the mixture into sweet moulds or, alternatively, line a tray with some cling film and pour your mixture in. If using, sprinkle the chopped goji berries over the chocolate.

Place the chocolate in the fridge for about 2 hours or in the freezer for about 20 minutes.

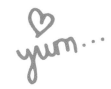

Grandad's Bikkies
(aka Homemade Fig Rolls)

My kids have grown up calling their grandad 'Grandad Bikkies' due to the fact that, every time they visit, he always gives them fig rolls. These little cookies are my healthy alternative to the regular store-bought kind and my next plan is to sneak them into Grandad's cupboard.

Makes 24 bikkies

180g dried figs (roughly 12 figs)

200ml fresh orange juice (about 3 oranges)

1 teaspoon vanilla extract

170g oat flour

2 puréed bananas

½ teaspoon baking powder

120g nut butter (I used almond)

60ml rapeseed oil

plain flour, for rolling

Preheat oven to 180°C/350°F/gas 4.

Put the figs, orange juice and vanilla into a saucepan. Place over a medium heat and, when it starts to bubble, lower the heat and simmer for 15 minutes until the figs start to break down and become lovely and soft. Then take the pan off the heat and leave aside to cool before puréeing the mixture in a blender.

To make the pastry, place the oat flour, bananas, baking powder, nut butter and rapeseed oil into a bowl and mix until fully combined. It should resemble a very soft dough. Turn out on a counter top sprinkled with flour and split the pastry into 4 parts to make it easier to roll.

Take one part of the pastry, sprinkle flour over it and rub the rolling pin with flour as well. Roll out into a long rectangle, about half a centimetre thick. Spread a quarter of the fig purée down the middle and then carefully fold both sides of the pastry over the purée so that they overlap each other and the purée is not visible. I used a spatula to help fold it over. The pastry is pretty forgiving so if it tears just press it back together. Flip the roll over so the folds are on the bottom and use your hands to shape it. Then cut the pastry into 6 biscuits. Roll out the remaining parts of the pastry and repeat.

Place the biscuits on a baking sheet lined with parchment paper and bake for 15 minutes. Allow to cool fully before serving. Store in an airtight container for up to a week.

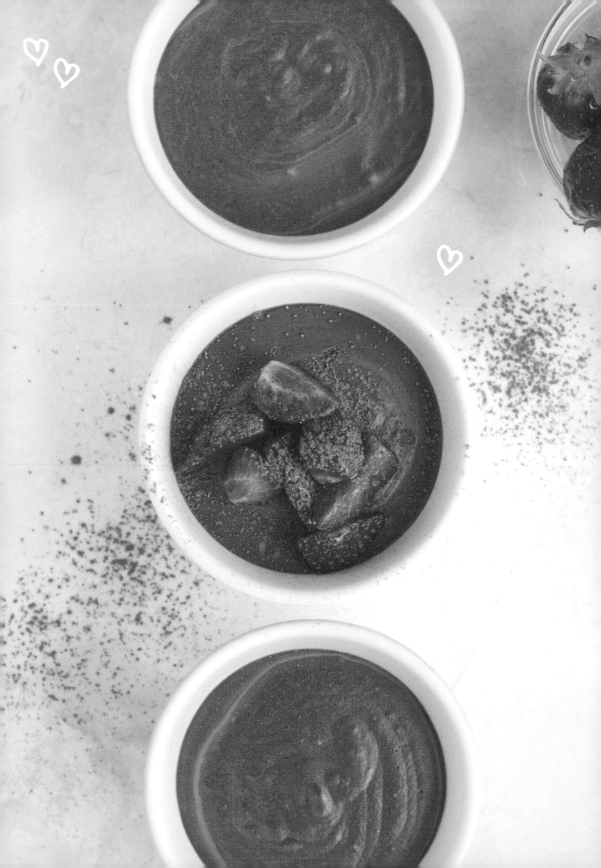

Chocolate
Mousse

If you have ever thought of giving up eating refined sugar then this is the dessert that will get you through. It is one of my absolute favourite things to eat and my little one's yummiest treat – smooth and creamy and just darn right chocolatey. It contains only 3 ingredients, takes less than 10 minutes to make and when refrigerated turns into the most decadent mousse. Serve with fresh strawberries for the ultimate dessert.

Serves 8

8 Medjool dates, pitted

400ml full-fat tinned coconut milk

4 tablespoons cacao powder

Add all of the ingredients to a blender. Blitz on high speed until the mixture becomes a smooth, silky chocolatey sauce.

Pour into ramekins and leave to set in the fridge overnight – it will magically turn into a delicious chocolate mousse!

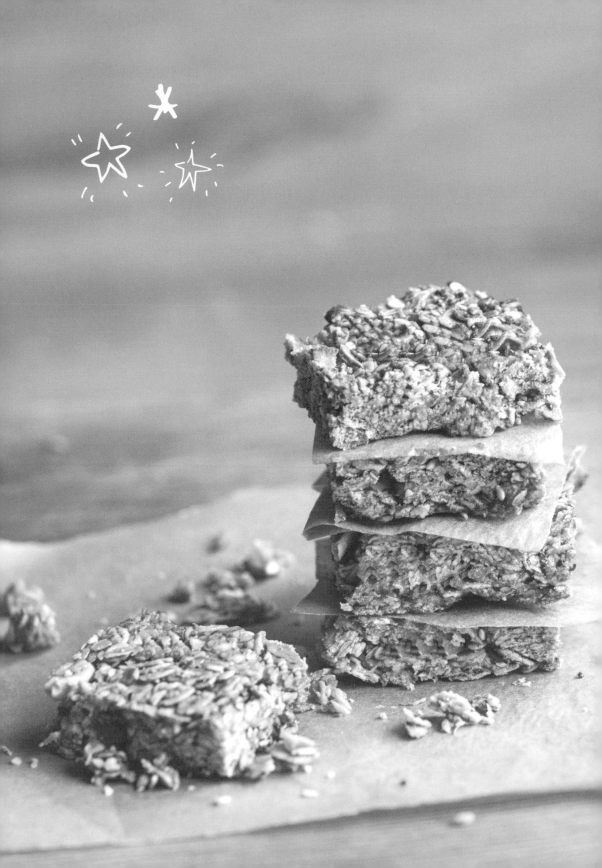

Toddler
Flapjacks

This recipe is one for older toddlers with teeth and is great for breakfast, as a snack or as a treat. We sometimes drizzle chocolate sauce over them to make them even yummier.

Makes 24 toddler bars

6 tbsp (120g): 72.6g free sugar
(24 servings) 3g each

240g oats

50g sesame seeds

75g pumpkin seeds

75g sunflower seeds

140g coconut oil

6 tablespoons maple syrup

120g almond or cashew butter

Preheat oven to 140°C/275°F/gas 1.

Place the oats and sesame seeds in a large bowl.

Use a pestle and mortar to grind the pumpkin and sunflower seeds until they resemble fine breadcrumbs and then add them to the bowl.

Melt the coconut oil with the maple syrup and pour over the oat mixture. Stir really well to make sure everything is coated with the oil. You can adjust the sweetness to your liking.

Pour the mixture into a 26 x 20cm baking tin lined with parchment paper. Then, using a spatula, spread the mixture evenly. Use a large spoon to press it down hard and really compress it.

Bake for 30 minutes and then remove from the oven. Leave to cool fully before slicing into 24 little bars.

Stores in an airtight container for a week.

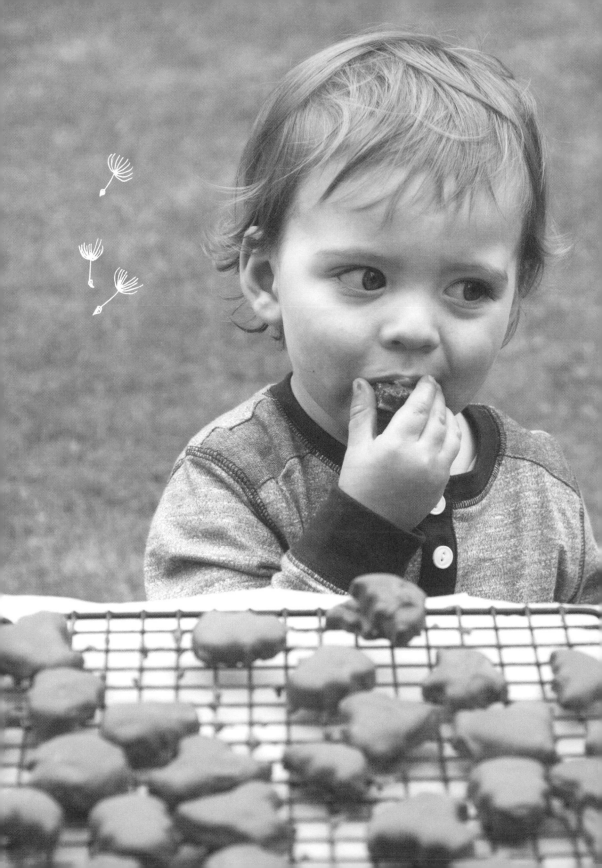

Baby Shortbread
Cookies

Yummy little cookies that are full to the brim with only nourishing ingredients. They are soft and easy for little hands to manage, and they taste so good that the only problem will be keeping them just for the baby!

Makes 24 cookies

125g Baby Chocolate: 12.1g free sugar (24 servings) 0.5g each

130g coconut flour

120g buckwheat flour

1 teaspoon baking powder

140g cashew butter

2 eggs

8 Medjool dates, soaked for 10 minutes in boiling water

2 teaspoons vanilla extract

125g Baby Chocolate (see page 236)

Preheat oven to 160°C/325°F/gas 3.

Place flours in a mixing bowl along with the baking powder. Add the cashew butter, eggs, dates and vanilla to a blender and blend into a purée.

Place this mixture in a separate bowl and then slowly add in the flour mixture until fully combined. If you have a mixer, you can use this rather than doing it by hand – or if you are like me and would like to build some muscle in your arms, do it the harder way. When the mixture resembles a dough, press it together, wrap in cling film and leave in the fridge for about an hour.

Split the dough into 2 parts to make it easier to roll out. Roll each piece to 5–7mm thick before cutting out the cookies with whatever cookie cutters you like.

Place on a baking tray lined with parchment paper and bake for 8–10 minutes or until golden. Because my cookies were quite small they cooked in 8 minutes. Watch them carefully and, when done, remove and place on a wire rack to cool.

Melt the chocolate in a bowl over a saucepan a quarter full of simmering water (make sure the water doesn't touch the base of the bowl). Dip the cookies in until they are completely covered.

Place on a plate lined with parchment paper and pop in the fridge to set.

Store in an airtight container for 4–5 days.

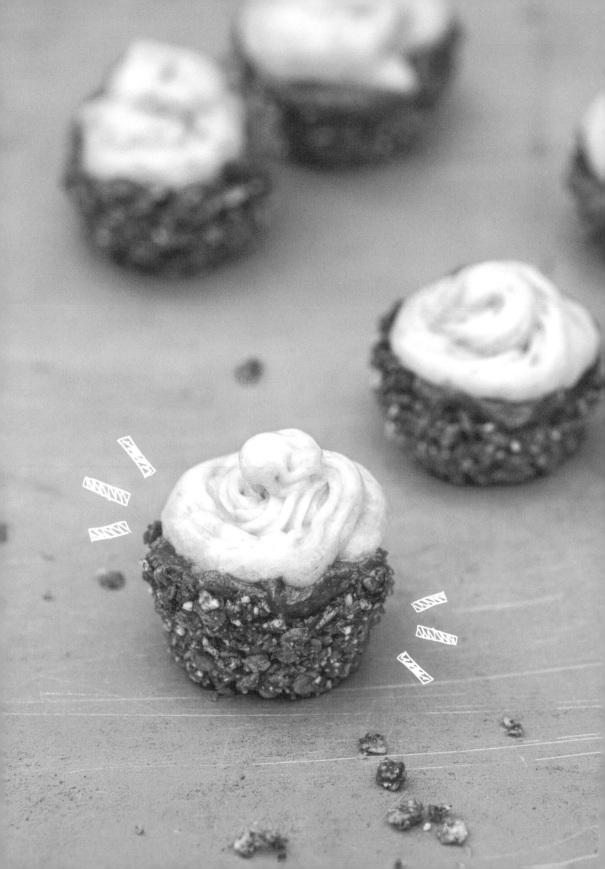

Banoffee Bites

Banoffee is one of those desserts that just screams indulgence. A rich caramel sauce poured over a crumbly biscuit base and topped with bananas and cream – as desserts go, it doesn't get any better. But because I don't eat sugary desserts any more, I have created the wonderful (and still very indulgent) banoffee bite. These can be eaten raw – however, baking the base slightly keeps them in shape, making them perfect for little hands.

Makes 24 bites

1 tbsp (20g) : 12.1g free sugar
(24 servings) 0.5g each

For the base

120g oats

70g sunflower seeds

70g pumpkin seeds

1 tablespoon maple syrup

4 tablespoons rapeseed oil

1 tablespoon cacao powder

For the caramel

6 Medjool dates

3 tablespoons cashew butter

2 tablespoons boiling water

For the banana nice-cream

4 bananas, peeled

4 tablespoons coconut cream

Preheat oven to 180°C/350°F/gas 4.

Add the oats, sunflower seeds and pumpkin seeds to a food processor and process until it resembles fine breadcrumbs. Add the maple syrup, rapeseed oil and cacao powder, and process again until it forms a dough.

Spoon a heaped teaspoon of the dough into a lightly oiled mini-muffin tin. Use a pestle to press the mixture down. When you have used up all the mixture, bake them in the oven for 12 minutes. Remove and leave to cool while you prepare the filling.

Add the Medjool dates, cashew butter and boiling water to a clean food processor and process until it comes together as a caramel sauce. If you need to add more water do so 1 tablespoon at a time. The sauce should be thick but smooth enough to fall off the spoon.

To make the banana nice-cream, place the bananas and coconut cream in a blender. Blend at a high speed until the bananas become a smooth, thick ice-cream texture.

To assemble the banoffee bites, spoon a teaspoon of the caramel onto each base, then add a heaped teaspoon of the banana nice-cream to the top.

Eat straight away or store in the freezer until you are ready to enjoy.

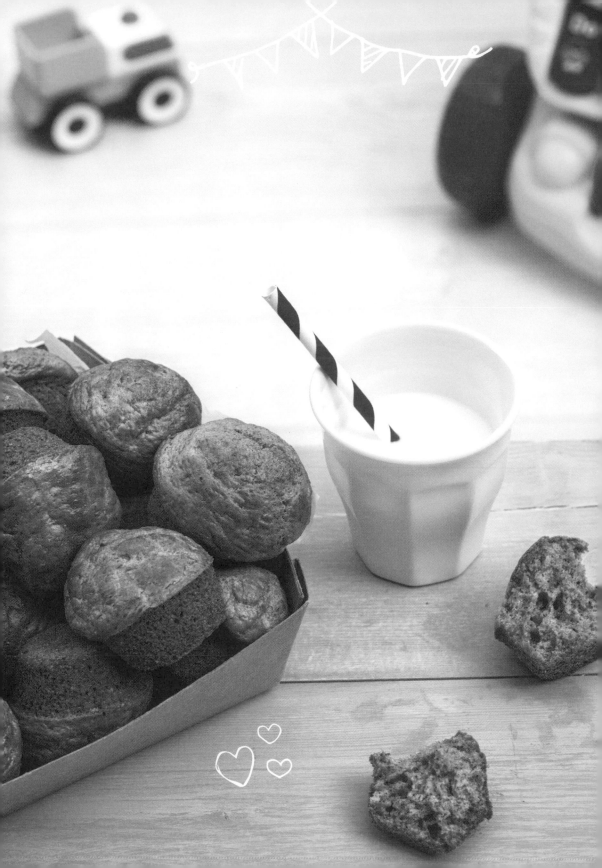

Carrot Cake
Mini-Muffins

Deliciously soft and moist, and packed with nutritious goodness, these muffins are really versatile and work great as a treat – as well as getting some extra veg into your little one's diet.

Makes 24

80ml: 96.8g free sugar
(24 servings) 4g each

300g plain flour

2 teaspoons baking powder

250ml milk

2 eggs

60ml rapeseed oil

1 teaspoon ground allspice

1 teaspoon ground cinnamon

80ml maple syrup

150g carrot, grated

2 teaspoons vanilla extract

Preheat oven to 200°C/400°F/gas 6.

Sieve flour and baking powder into a large mixing bowl.

In a jug, whisk together the milk, eggs and rapeseed oil. Make a well in the centre of the flour and slowly whisk the wet mixture in until it forms a smooth batter.

Add the spices, maple syrup, carrot and vanilla and give everything a good stir.

Spoon the mixture into an oiled mini-muffin tin.

Bake for 25 minutes until the muffins have risen and are golden brown – if you stick a toothpick into them it should come out clean.

Serve warm or cold. Keeps in an airtight container for up to a week.

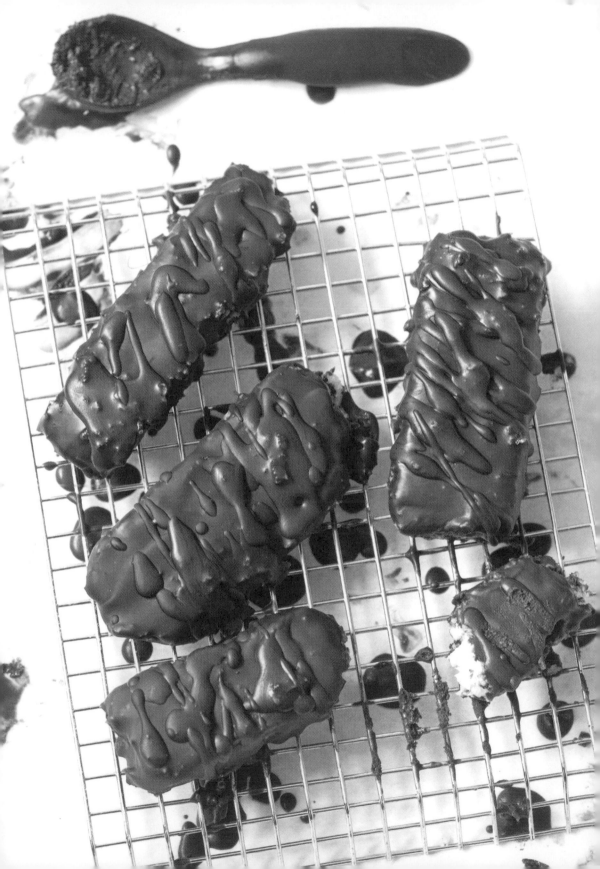

Coconut
Chocolate Bars

Bounty bars are my ultimate chocolate treat and I was determined to make a healthy version of them. These bars are refined-sugar free and are all types of good. Store in the freezer, as the coconut stays soft, which also makes them ideal for teething baby gums.

Makes 12

6 tbsp (120g): 72.6g free sugar
(12 servings) 6g each

For the filling

80g sugar-free desiccated coconut

2 tablespoons coconut oil, melted

3 tablespoons maple syrup

1 tablespoon vanilla extract

2 tablespoons coconut cream (the thick cream on top of coconut milk)

For the chocolate

50g cacao butter

3 tablespoons cacao powder

3 tablespoons maple syrup

Preheat oven to 200°C/400°F/gas 6.

Spread the desiccated coconut on a large baking tray and place into the hot oven for about 15 minutes. It should start to turn slightly crispy. This gives it a lovely, toasted taste. Remove from the oven and place into a bowl.

Add the coconut oil, maple syrup, vanilla extract and coconut cream and mix until fully combined. Place into a 26 x 20cm baking tin lined with cling film. Press down hard all across the mixture to compact it, then cover and freeze for about 2 hours.

After this time, melt the cacao butter in a bowl over a quarter-full pot of simmering water. Make sure the water doesn't touch the bowl. Once melted, remove from the heat. Gently whisk in the cacao powder, sweeten with maple syrup and leave in the fridge for up to 5 mins to thicken slightly.

Remove the coconut filling from the freezer and take out of the tin. Cut into 12 pieces, then dip each one into the chocolate to fully coat. Place onto a tray lined with parchment paper and drizzle over any remaining chocolate.

Store in the fridge for up to 1 week.

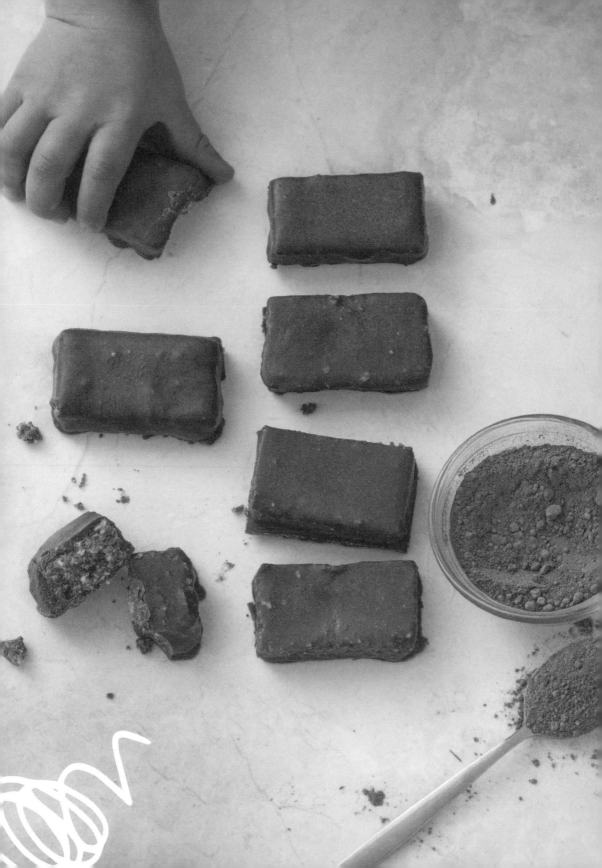

Raw Snickers Bites

A deliciously smooth and healthy take on one of my favourite childhood treats, these super-quick no-bake bars are full of nutty goodness and a winner with kids of all ages.

Makes 24

1 tbsp (20g): 12.1g free sugar
(24 servings) 0.5g each

For the filling

8 Medjool dates

65g coconut oil, melted

60g ground almonds

3 teaspoons vanilla extract

70g smooth peanut butter

1 tablespoon cacao powder

50g oats

For the chocolate coating

50g cacao butter

1 tablespoon maple syrup

1 teaspoon sugar-free vanilla extract

1 tablespoon cacao powder

1 tablespoon cashew butter (or other smooth nut butter)

1 tablespoon tahini

Add all of the filling ingredients to a food processor and whizz until they form a ball.

Pour into a 20 x 20cm tin lined with parchment paper and then, using the back of a spoon, press down until it is uniformly flattened. Cover the tin with cling film and place in the fridge for 4 hours until set.

To make the chocolate, bring a saucepan of water, roughly a quarter full, to a boil and then reduce to a simmer. Add the cacao butter to a glass bowl and place over the water to melt. Make sure the water doesn't touch the bowl. When melted, remove from the heat and stir in the remaining ingredients until it becomes smooth and silky. Leave the chocolate in a cool place for about 5 minutes so that it can thicken up. This makes it easier to coat the bars.

Cut into 24 pieces. Dip each into the sauce and then place on a flat baking tray lined with parchment paper. When you are finished, place in the fridge to set for about 10 minutes. If the chocolate is too thin, you can repeat the dipping.

To re-melt the chocolate, place it back over the saucepan of water for a few moments and then re-dip the bars.

Store in the fridge for 1 week.

Raw Seed
and Oat Bars

Seeds are nutritional powerhouses and a great way to get some extra vitamins and minerals into children, especially when they are going through a fussy stage. These bars are full of goodness and make a great treat for the weekends.

Makes 12

1 tbsp (20g) : 12.1g free sugar
(12 servings) 1g each

For the seed bars

8 Medjool dates

4 tablespoons tahini

160g smooth peanut butter

130g coconut oil, melted

1 teaspoon vanilla extract

200g oats

50g pumpkin seeds

50g sunflower seeds

2 tablespoons chia seeds

For the chocolate

50g cacao butter

1 tablespoon cacao powder

1 tablespoon maple syrup

1 tablespoon tahini

1 tablespoon cashew butter

1 teaspoon vanilla extract

Add the dates, tahini, peanut butter, coconut oil and vanilla to a blender and blend until smooth and creamy. Pour into a bowl.

Add the remaining seed-bar ingredients and stir well. Pour into a small tray lined with parchment paper and press down with the back of a spoon to compact.

To make the chocolate, add the cacao butter to a bowl and place over a saucepan a quarter full of simmering water. Make sure the water doesn't touch the bowl. Remove from the heat when fully melted.

Whisk in the cacao powder, maple syrup, tahini, cashew butter and vanilla until it becomes smooth and silky. Then pour over the seed bars.

Leave to set in the fridge for at least 4 hours (or in the freezer for about 30 minutes if you can't wait).

Cut into 12 pieces and store in an airtight container for about 1 week.

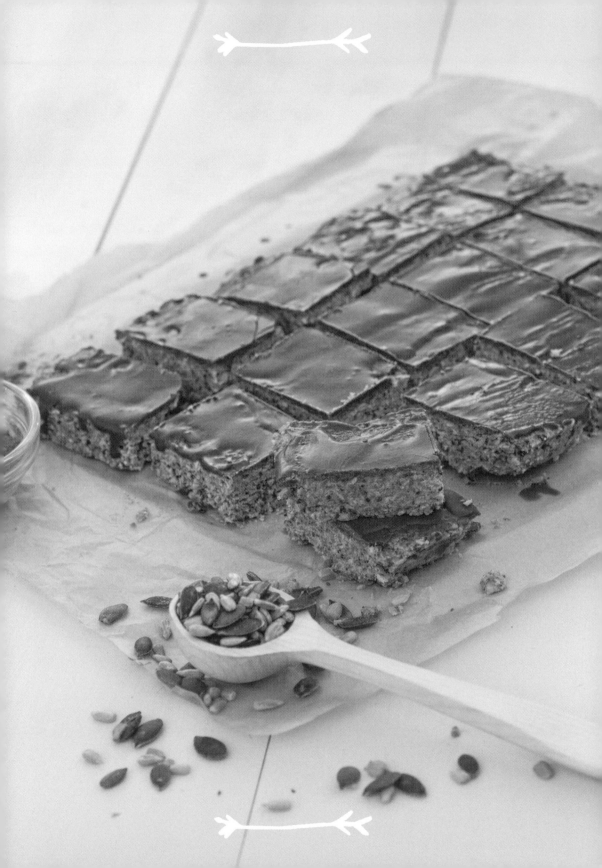

Coconut Macaroons

One bite of these soft, melt-in-your-mouth macaroons will bring you back to your childhood. This is my healthy take on these normally sugar-filled treats, packed with only nourishing ingredients you won't mind giving your baby.

Makes 12

125g Baby Chocolate: 12.1g free sugar
(12 servings) 1g each

250g grated coconut or unsweetened desiccated coconut

3 pitted Medjool dates

½ orange, juice only

2 tablespoons coconut oil

1 teaspoon orange-blossom water or vanilla extract

2 egg whites

125g Baby Chocolate (see page 236)

Preheat oven to 160°C/325°F/gas 3.

Toast the coconut by placing it on a tray and baking for about 15 minutes. This helps release that delicious coconut-y flavour.

Meanwhile, place the Medjool dates, orange juice and coconut oil in a saucepan and gently heat, stirring all the time. Once the mixture starts to bubble, turn the heat to low and keep stirring until the dates start to break up and dissolve, turning it into a sticky caramel mixture.

Take off the heat, add the orange-blossom water and allow the mixture to cool. Add the toasted coconut and mix well.

Whisk the egg whites until they are light and fluffy and forming stiff peaks. This only takes about a minute or so. Fold the egg whites into the coconut mixture and, when it is completely combined, use an ice-cream scoop to place portions of the mixture onto a baking sheet lined with parchment paper.

Bake for 15–20 minutes or until they start to brown, and then remove from the oven and leave on a wire rack to cool.

Melt the chocolate in a bowl over a saucepan a quarter full of simmering water. Be careful not to let the water touch the bottom of the bowl.

Drizzle the melted chocolate over the macaroons – if you like, you can dip the base into the chocolate also.

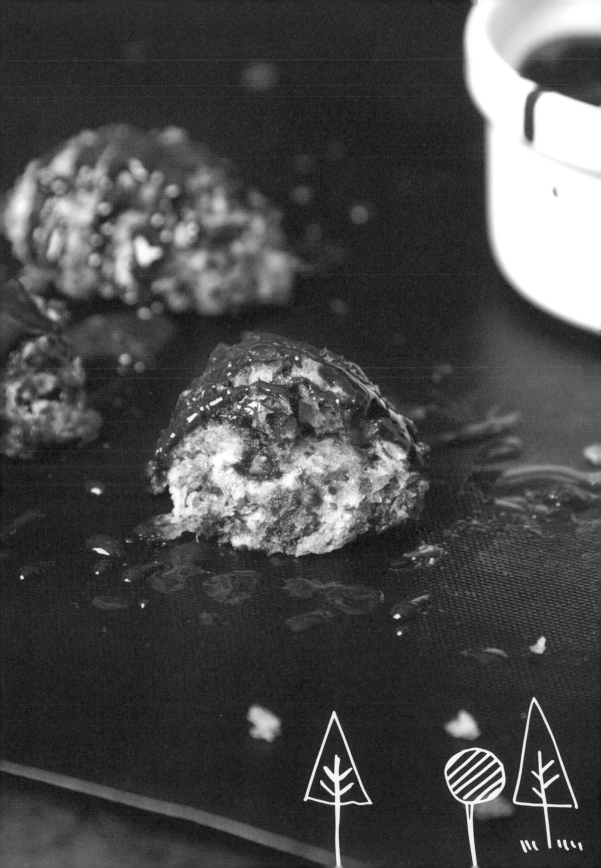

Raw Avocado
Key Lime Pies

Cashews are such amazing nuts. Soaked overnight, then drained and blended, they magically turn into a creamy, silky mixture. Cashew cream can be used to replace sour cream, if your little one is dairy free. It can also be used to make fabulous desserts like these yummy Key lime pies. They taste almost like cheese cake yet they are refined-sugar and dairy free, and the best part is that they get their lovely green colour from avocado and spinach – don't tell the kids because they'll never guess!

Makes 24 mini-pies

For the base

3 Medjool dates, soaked in boiling water for 10 minutes

80g oats

70g pecans

50g ground almonds

1 teaspoon vanilla extract

3 tablespoons coconut oil, melted

For the filling

135g cashews, soaked overnight

1 ripe avocado

2 limes, zest and juice

2 tablespoons maple syrup

30g baby spinach leaves

2 tablespoons coconut oil, melted

natural yogurt, to top
1 lime, sliced thinly and cut into 24 wedges

Drain the Medjool dates and add them and all the ingredients for the base to a food processor. Blend until it forms a ball of dough. Remove and divide into 24 evenly sized pieces.

Place 24 mini-muffin cases in a mini-muffin tin and add a piece of dough to each one, using your fingers to flatten them.

To make the filling, drain the cashews and place them in a food processor. They take around 10 minutes to become smooth, silky and creamy and should have no grainy, nutty parts remaining.

Add the remaining filling ingredients to the food processor and blend until totally combined.

Spoon the filling into the mini-muffin cases until it comes to the top of each one. When you are finished, top each one with a little natural yogurt and a tiny wedge of lime. Place in the fridge for at least 4 hours until set.

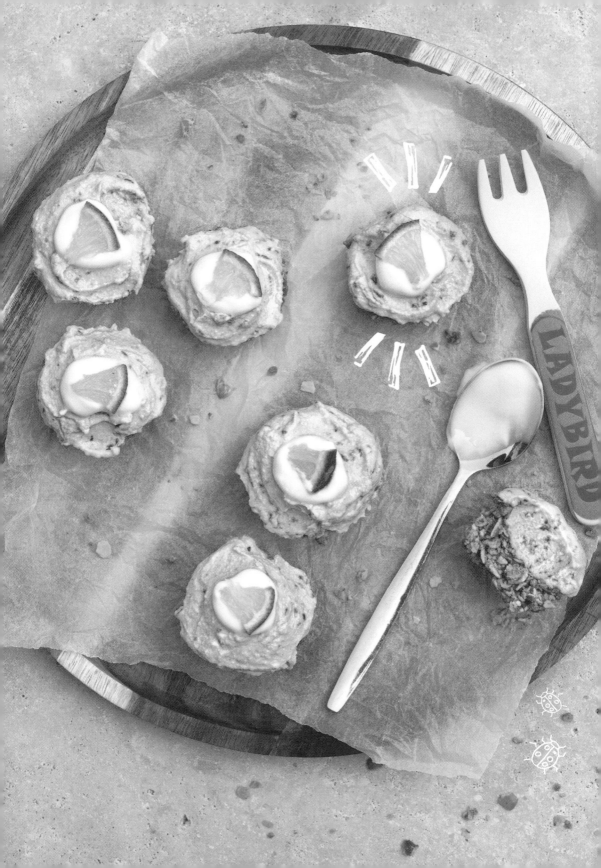

Toddler
Veggie Crisps

Veggie crisps are a brilliant toddler snack. I don't cook mine until they are completely crispy so they are easy for little mouths to manage. This is such a simple recipe and they taste so delicious you will cook them again and again for your family.

Serves 2 adults and 2 children

2 medium-sized raw beetroot, scrubbed and finely sliced

4 medium carrots, scrubbed and finely sliced

2 parsnips, scrubbed and finely sliced

3 tablespoons rapeseed oil

sprig rosemary, leaves picked and finely chopped

Preheat oven to 190°C/375°F/gas 5.

Place the sliced vegetables in separate bowls, as the carrot and beetroot will discolour the parsnip.

Add 1 tablespoon of rapeseed oil and a third of the rosemary to each bowl and then, using your hands, mix it through the slices of vegetables to make sure they are totally covered.

Spread the slices onto trays lined with parchment paper, making sure they have a little space around them and that none of them are overlapping.

Bake for 25 minutes for soft vegetable crisps.

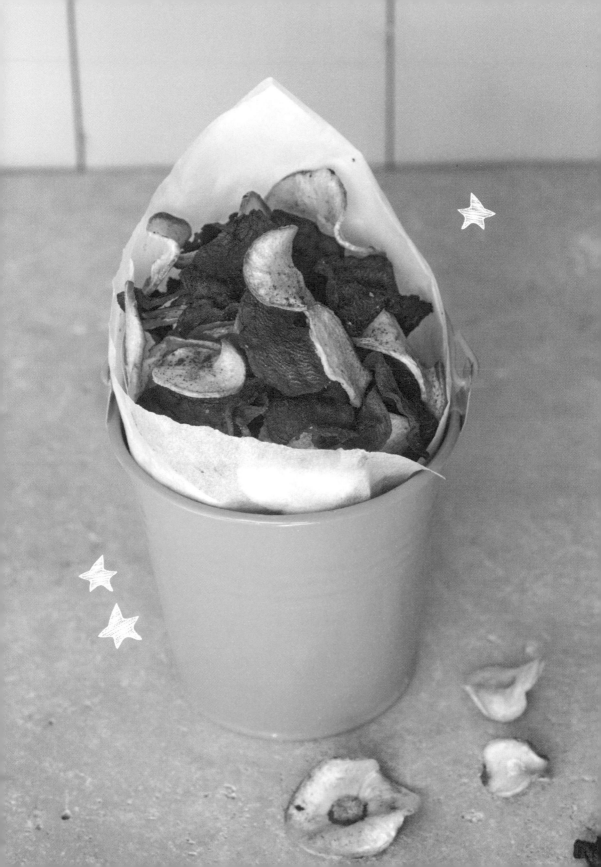

YIPPEE!
Let's Have a
PARTY
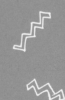

Celebrations and treats

go hand in hand, and these recipes are not only
healthy and nutritious but also easy to make
– just perfect for when you have a group of
little ones coming to party on down!

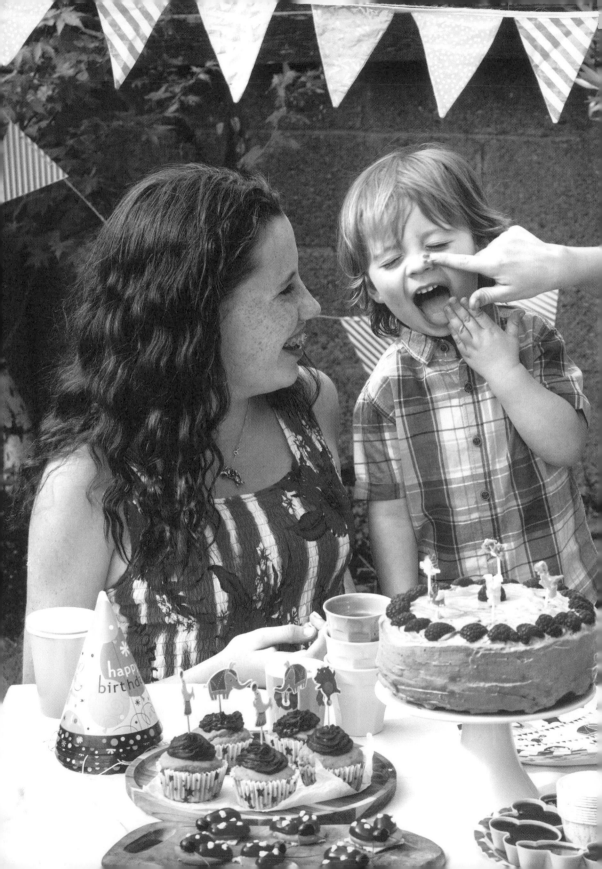

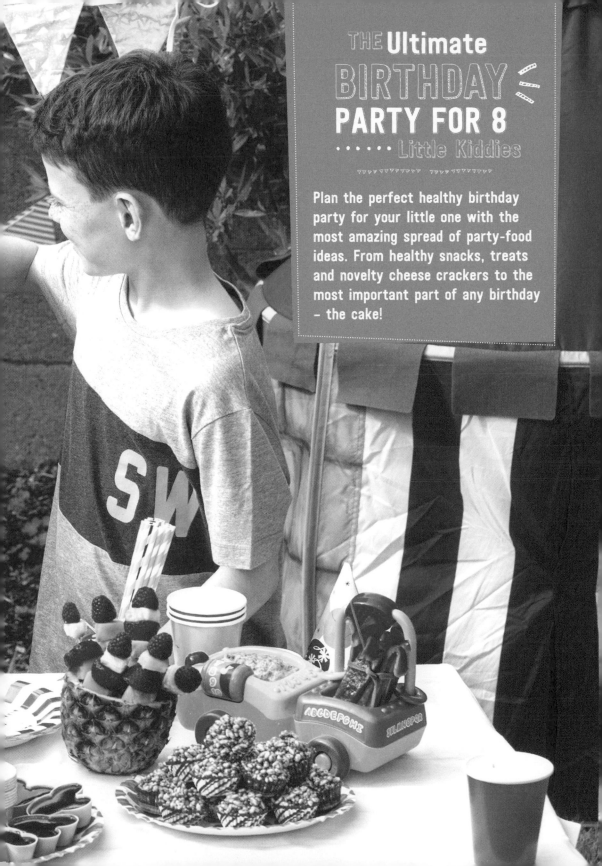

THE Ultimate BIRTHDAY PARTY FOR 8
····· Little Kiddies

Plan the perfect healthy birthday party for your little one with the most amazing spread of party-food ideas. From healthy snacks, treats and novelty cheese crackers to the most important part of any birthday – the cake!

Healthy and Yummy
Baby Crispie Buns

Spooning this mixture into the little paper cups immediately brought me back to being a 10-year-old girl. I think crispie buns are a standard when it comes to kids' parties so in true Baby-Led-Feeding style I have substituted my own delicious homemade chocolate for the regular sugary version and organic wholegrain puffed rice and puffed quinoa from a local health store for the sugary cereal. Yes, these may be a standard party treat but if your little ones gobble up this version, you will be smiling from ear to ear. Happy goodness!

Makes 24 mini-buns

250g Baby Chocolate: 24.2g free sugar
20g Baby Fine Granola: 1.5g
(24 servings) 1.07g each

250g Baby Chocolate (see page 236)

80g naturally puffed wholegrain rice

30g puffed quinoa

12g milled linseeds

12g milled chia seeds

20g Baby Fine Granola (see page 42)

Melt the chocolate in a bowl over a saucepan a quarter full of simmering water (ensuring the water doesn't touch the bottom of the bowl). When the chocolate has melted, remove it from the heat immediately, as you don't want to ruin its good properties.

Place all of the remaining ingredients in a large bowl, pour the chocolate over and give a good stir until everything has been covered in chocolate.

Spoon into a mini-muffin tin lined with mini-muffin cases (any leftover mixture can be divided between regular muffin cases for older children) and leave in the fridge to set for about 1 hour.

Pineapple and Cherry
Jelly and Nice-Cream

Wibbly, wobbly, deliciously healthy jelly on a plate. Jelly is one of those desserts loved by children of all ages, and just hearing the words 'jelly and ice-cream' immediately brings me back to childhood memories. I wanted to make a healthy version for my little ones – with absolutely no added sugars – and I discovered that pineapple is the best sweet fruit to use as a base. It works so well to make this jelly a totally yummy kiddie treat.

Makes 8 portions

300g pineapple flesh, roughly chopped

300g cherries, stones in

150ml water

1½ tablespoons grass-fed gelatine

8 sliced bananas, frozen

Place the pineapple and cherries in a saucepan with the water and bring to the boil. Simmer with the lid on for 15 minutes. Then, using a masher, mash the fruit so that it breaks apart and becomes watery and mushy.

Place a sieve over a medium-sized bowl, pour the fruit into the sieve and use the masher to gently push it through until all the liquid runs into the bowl. Pour the juice back into the saucepan and place over a very low heat.

Place the gelatine into a cup and add 4 tablespoons of cold water. Stir well and leave to bloom for about 2 minutes. Then add it to the warm fruit liquid and stir well until totally dissolved.

Pour the jelly into little moulds and leave in the fridge to set for at least 2 hours.

To serve, take the frozen bananas out of the freezer and add to a blender. Blend until smooth and creamy. Spoon a little banana nice-cream on top of each jelly and serve.

yum!

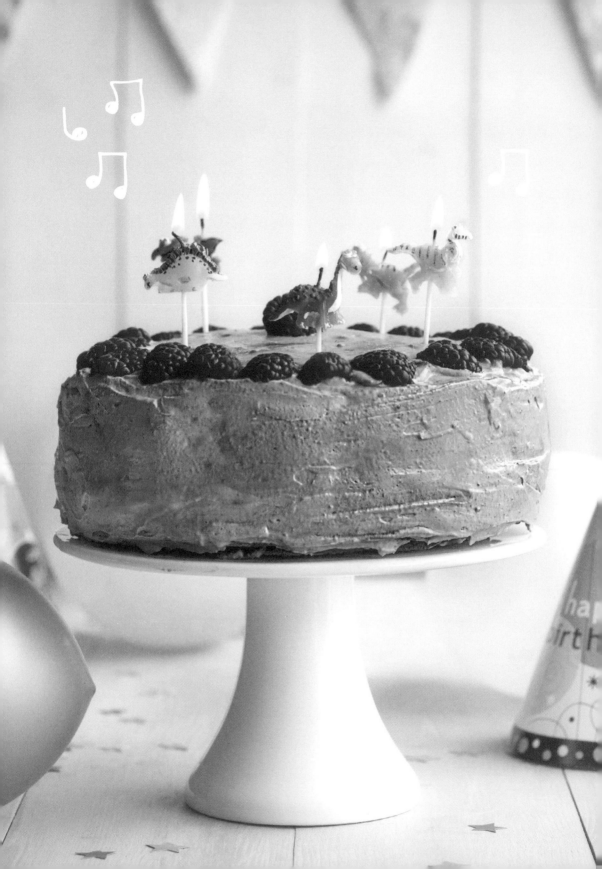

Raspberry Frosting
Birthday Cake

Using sweet potato in cake may sound a little odd, but I promise it doesn't taste anything like something you would eat for dinner instead of dessert. This cake is deliciously light with a spongey, pillow-y texture.

Serves 12

160mls: 96.8g free sugar
(12 servings) 8.06g each

For the cake

160g buckwheat flour

40g coconut flour

2 teaspoons baking powder

3 eggs

250ml Easy Apple Sauce
(see page 193)

200g cooked sweet potato,
puréed

2 tablespoons cacao
powder

80ml maple syrup

For the raspberry jam

125g raspberries

2 tablespoons water

2 tablespoons maple syrup

4 tablespoons chia seeds

For the raspberry frosting

280g cream cheese

1 tablespoon vanilla
extract

125g raspberries

2 tablespoons maple syrup

extra raspberries, to
decorate

Preheat oven to 180°C/350°F/gas 4.

Place flours and baking powder in a bowl and leave aside.

In a separate bowl, add the eggs, apple sauce, sweet potato, cacao and maple syrup and, using an electric whisk if you have one, beat until the mixture is lovely and creamy. Slowly whisk in the flour, little by little, until fully combined.

Divide the mixture equally between two 22cm springform tins lined with parchment paper and bake for 30 minutes. You will know the cake is cooked when a skewer comes out clean. Remove from the tin and leave to cool fully on a wire rack before assembling.

Meanwhile, add the raspberries and water to a saucepan and bring to the boil. Stir well and reduce the heat to medium. When the raspberries have become mushy, add the maple syrup and chia seeds. Cook for another few minutes until the jam has thickened,.and then remove from the heat and leave to cool.

To make the frosting, beat the cream cheese with the vanilla until it is light and fluffy. In a separate bowl, mash the raspberries with the maple syrup until they become smooth and silky. Then add them to the cream cheese and beat until it has turned beautiful and pink.

To decorate, spread the raspberry chia jam on top of one of the cakes then sit the other cake on top. Scoop the cream cheese frosting onto the cake and, using a spatula, spread all over until the cake is totally covered. Decorate the top with fresh raspberries before serving.

Baby Cupcakes
with Beetroot Frosting

It wouldn't be a birthday party without a cupcake or fairy cake! These are lovely, light and fluffy and just the perfect size for little hands. They also work as a cupcake birthday cake if you stack them, and each one is a little child's portion. I bought beetroot powder for the frosting in my local health-food store but you can make it by cooking slices of beetroot in the oven until they are totally dried out and then using a pestle and mortar to grind them into powder. You can also try different vegetables, like spinach and carrot, for other colours.

Makes 24 mini-cupcakes (or 12 regular)

3 tbsp (60g): 36.3g free sugar
(24 servings) 1.5g each

For the cupcakes

180g cooked sweet potato, puréed

125ml milk

75ml rapeseed oil

2 tablespoons maple syrup

1 teaspoon vanilla extract

1 egg

150g plain white flour

120g buckwheat flour

1 teaspoon baking powder

1 egg white

For the frosting

400ml tinned full-fat coconut milk (chilled in the fridge for 4 hours or, preferably, overnight)

½ teaspoon beetroot powder

1 tablespoon maple syrup

Preheat oven to 180°C/350°F/gas 4.

Add the sweet potato, milk, oil, maple syrup, vanilla and 1 egg to a food processor and process until light and airy. Mix the flours and baking powder and add slowly, a few spoons at a time, until it has been fully combined. You can also do this by hand with a wooden spoon.

In a separate bowl whisk the egg white until light and fluffy. Then fold in the sweet potato mixture – don't over-mix, as you want to keep it light and airy.

Divide the mixture into a mini-muffin tin lined with mini-muffin cases. Bake for 25 minutes until they are firm to the touch.

Remove from the oven and cool on a wire rack while you make the frosting.

Remove the tin of coconut milk from the fridge and scoop out the coconut cream (the set part only). Add to a bowl and whisk until stiff peaks form. Whisk in the beetroot power and sweeten to your taste with the maple syrup.

Use a piping bag to pipe the coconut cream on top of the cupcakes and then serve.

Fruit Skewers

These little sticks of fruit look very cute and, funnily enough, are always the first thing the smaller kids go for at parties. I kept the pineapple shell and served them in that for an extra bit of fun.

Makes 8

2 kiwis, each peeled and cut into 4

1 mango, peeled, stoned and cut into large chunks

½ pineapple, peeled, cored and cut into large chunks

4 strawberries, halved

8 raspberries

8 ice-pop sticks

Push a piece of each chopped fruit onto each stick, leaving enough room at the end for a little hand to hold. Top the stick with an upside-down raspberry. Serve cool.

Bug Bites

This isn't really a recipe so much as a cute way to serve cheese and crackers for a kids' birthday party.

Makes 8

8 oat crackers

8 slices cheddar cheese, cut into circles

8 plum cherry tomatoes, halved

8 chive tips

4 blueberries, halved

1 teaspoon sour cream or Greek yogurt

Put the crackers on a serving plate. Add a circle of cheese to each one and then place 2 cherry tomatoes halves, cut side down, side by side and spread a little apart at the end, to make the wings.

Place two chive tips, sticking out, where the two halves of the tomato meet (for the antennae) and hold them down with half a blueberry (for the head).

Use the tip of a sharp knife to add 3 little blobs of sour cream or Greek yogurt to each tomato half to make spots for your bugs' wings.

THE Ultimate HALLOWEEN PARTY FOR 8 ···· Little Kiddies

My kiddies love Halloween

and having a party at home is the best craic ever, with ghoulish,
creepy, scary foods that they just giggle over with excitement.
These treats are all sugar free and there are a few savoury ones
too to fill their tummies up with goodness before they start
on their haul of goodies.

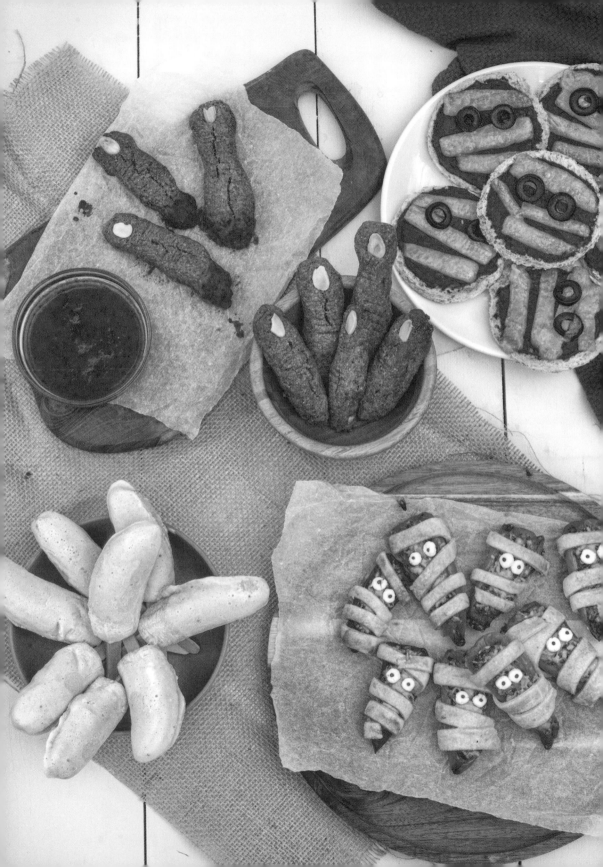

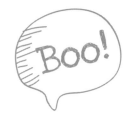

Stuffed Mummy Peppers

These baby peppers are frighteningly good and are the perfect little food to have on a party table as they are both delicious and full of goodness.

Makes 16

100g plain flour

30g unsalted butter

3–4 tablespoons of water

8 heaped teaspoons of cooked couscous, brown rice, bulgur wheat or quinoa

1 handful fresh spinach leaves, chopped

2 tablespoons parsley leaves, chopped

1 clove garlic, crushed

½ lemon, juice only

2 tablespoons olive oil

black pepper, to season

8 baby peppers

60g cheddar cheese, grated

1 egg, beaten

1 tablespoon goat's cheese

32 mustard seeds or 2 olives, finely chopped

Preheat oven to 180°C/350°F/gas 4.

Add the flour to a bowl and, using your hands, rub in the butter until the mixture resembles fine breadcrumbs. Add the water 1 tablespoon at a time until the pastry comes together. Turn onto a floured surface and roll into a thin rectangle. Cut into 16 long, skinny strips.

Place the grain (I used bulgur wheat) in a bowl and add the spinach leaves, parsley, garlic, lemon juice and olive oil. Season with a little black pepper.

Cut and deseed the peppers then fill each half with the mixture. Sprinkle over the cheddar, put the peppers onto a tray and place in the oven for about 5 minutes until the cheese melts (this makes it easier to wrap the pastry without the cheese falling off.)

Take the tray out of the oven and allow to cool to the touch. Then take a strip of the pastry and wrap around each pepper similar to a mummy's bandage.

Using a clean paintbrush or pastry brush, paint the pastry with the beaten egg.

Bake in the oven for 15 minutes.

To serve, add 2 little eyes to each pepper by rolling a tiny piece of goat's cheese in your hand then pressing it flat. Add a mustard seed or a tiny piece of olive to each eye for pupils.

Serve warm.

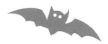

Mummy Pizza Toast

The quickest pizzas you will ever make and kids love them. I cook these when we have a lot of kids to feed and don't want to go to the trouble of making dough. Adding some olive eyes and cheese bandages to the toppings make the scary – but delicious – mummy faces!

Makes 8

8 slices homemade wholegrain bread

4 tablespoons unsalted tomato purée

1 garlic clove, crushed

4 tablespoons water

pepper, to season

8 slices cheddar cheese, each cut into 3 strips

2 black olives, each cut into 4 circular slices

Cut the slices of bread into circles using a large cookie cutter. Lightly toast each side.

Add the tomato purée, garlic, water and pepper to a bowl and stir well to make the sauce.

Spread some tomato sauce onto one side of each slice of toast, and arrange three strips of cheese on top. Put two olive slices on for eyes and serve!

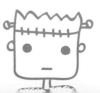

Banana Ghost Pops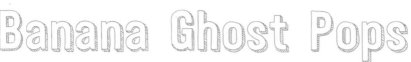

Ghoulish banana pops that are not only healthy but also a yummy treat –
especially for teething babies.

Makes 8 Portions

9 bananas

250g yogurt

1 teaspoon vanilla extract

8 ice-pop sticks

Cut 8 of the bananas in half and push an ice-pop stick
into the thick end of each half. Place on a tray lined with
parchment paper and pop in the freezer until frozen – this
takes about 4 hours.

When the bananas are frozen, place the remaining banana,
yogurt and vanilla in a blender and blend into a smooth
purée.

Dip each banana into the yogurt mixture then replace on the
lined tray and refreeze for about an hour before repeating
again.

Store in the freezer until you are ready to serve.

Ghostly Severed Fingers

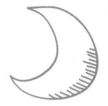

A very creepy treat that will delight kids of all ages – oat fingers, made with only healthy ingredients, dipped in blood ... I mean, raspberry jam!

Makes 16 fingers

4 tbsp (80g): 48.4g free sugar
(16 servings) 3g each

120g oat flour

2 puréed bananas

½ teaspoon baking powder

120g nut butter (I used almond)

60ml rapeseed oil

2 tablespoons maple syrup

16 flaked almonds

For the 'blood'

80g raspberries

80g cranberries

2 tablespoons maple syrup

Preheat oven to 180°C/350°F/gas 4.

Put the oat flour, bananas, baking powder, nut butter and rapeseed oil into a bowl and stir until fully combined. You can also use a food processor to make your job a little easier. It should resemble a very soft dough.

Take about one tablespoon of the mixture in your hand and roll into a long finger shape. Use your thumb to press down at the top to make a fingernail shape and use a knife to add lines on the knuckles.

Place on a baking tray lined with parchment paper and put a flaked almond into the indent for the fingernail.

Tear off a tiny piece from the end of each finger for dramatic effect. Bake in the oven for 12 minutes.

For the 'blood' (yummy jam), add the raspberries, cranberries and maple syrup to a blender and blend until smooth and silky. Serve in a bowl with the fingers. Remove the flaked almond before serving to little babies.

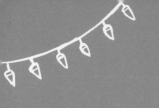

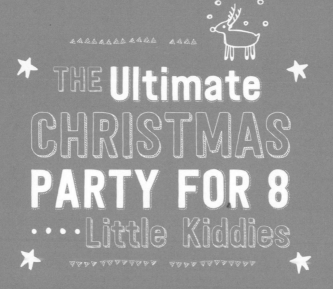

THE Ultimate CHRISTMAS PARTY FOR 8
····Little Kiddies

Give me Christmas
over any other time of the year - I just love it.
The joy and the love from everyone always brings
a tear to my eye. These recipes are great for when you
have friends with kids calling over and you want to
impress with a delicious, healthy spread.

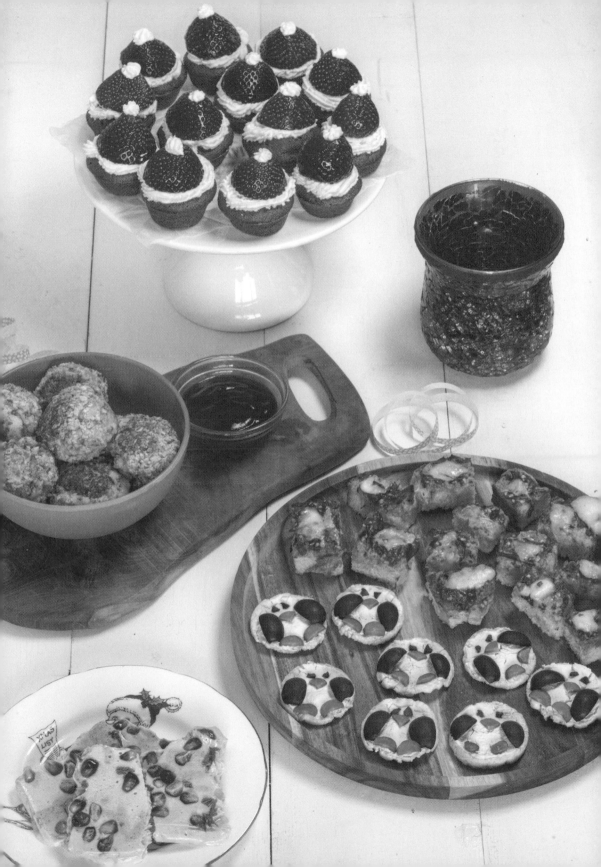

Christmas
Santa Brownies

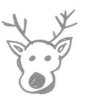

At Christmas, nothing beats a warm, gooey brownie, topped with coconut whipped cream and a strawberry hat. Delicious little Santas that taste as good as they look and the best part is that all the ingredients are nourishing. Good-for-you brownies – sure why wouldn't you let your little one have another?

Makes 24 mini-brownies

5 tbsp (100g): 60.7g free sugar
(24 servings) 2.5g each

For the brownies

120g coconut oil

4 tablespoons maple syrup

1 orange, zest of whole orange and juice of ½

2 teaspoons orange-blossom water or vanilla extract

2 tablespoons cacao powder

80g buckwheat flour

1 teaspoon baking powder

2 eggs

For the cream

400ml tinned full-fat coconut milk, refrigerated overnight

1 tablespoon maple syrup

24 strawberries

Preheat oven to 180°C/350°F/gas 4.

Place a large bowl over a saucepan a quarter full with water and put over a medium heat.

Add the coconut oil, maple syrup, orange zest and juice, orange blossom or vanilla extract and stir until fully melted.

Take off the heat and whisk in the cacao powder, buckwheat flour and baking powder. When it is smooth and silky, whisk the 2 eggs into the mixture.

Divide into a well-oiled mini-muffin tin and bake for 15 minutes. A skewer should come out clean when they are done. Leave on a wire tray to cool.

Meanwhile, carefully open the coconut milk, making sure not to shake it. Gently scoop out the coconut cream and place in a large bowl along with the maple syrup.

Using an electric whisk, beat until light and fluffy.

Use a piping bag to pipe a little coconut cream on top of the brownies. Place a strawberry upside down on top of it and, finally, pipe a tiny bit more of the coconut cream on top of the strawberry hat as a pompom.

Mint Yogurt Bark

Creamy frozen yogurt decorated with yummy Christmassy fruit. So easy and quick to make and little kiddies love it.

500g natural yogurt

4 bananas

1 tablespoon vanilla extract

3 tablespoons peppermint leaves, finely chopped

1 pomegranate, seeds only

Add the yogurt, banana and vanilla to a blender and blend until smooth and creamy.

Pour three-quarters of the mixture onto a tray lined with cling film. Add 2 tablespoons of the mint leaves to the remaining quarter and blend again until fully combined.

Drizzle this over the tin in a zig-zag pattern to get a minty drizzle everywhere.

Sprinkle the pomegranate seeds over it. Then sprinkle over the remaining mint leaves and freeze for about 4 hours. Break apart and serve.

Store in the freezer.

Penguin Crackers

Kids always tend to go for the sweet things first so simple crackers made into adorable animals work really well when you want them to be the first things eaten.

Makes 8

8 mini organic rice cakes

2 tablespoons soft goat's cheese

2 baby carrots, finely sliced

3 olives, 2 quartered and 1 finely chopped

Spread the goat's cheese on one side of each rice cake.

Take 2 slices of carrot and cut into quarters to make the beaks. Cut 8 slices in half to make the feet. Arrange one beak and two feet on each rice cake.

Place one olive quarter on each side of each cracker to make the wings. Place two pieces of chopped olive above each beak for the eyes, and serve.

Baby
Bruschetta Bites

A Christmas-inspired snack that is easy to make and tastes wonderful. I buy a natural rosemary and onion bread in our local French baker that contains only bread, yeast, rosemary, onion and olive oil. Delicious and really baby friendly.

Serves 2 adults and 2 children

4 slices good quality bread

1 clove garlic, peeled and cut in half

4 cherry tomatoes, finely chopped

2 tablespoons olive oil

4 basil leaves, finely chopped

40g buffalo mozzarella, finely chopped

Lightly toast the bread and cut off any crusts that would be too hard for little ones' gums. Gently rub one side of each piece of toasted bread with the cut side of a garlic half.

Heat the cherry tomatoes in a pan with the olive oil. Mash with a fork to make it lovely and saucy. Then remove from the heat and place the slices of bread onto the tomato – press them down to make sure they soak up all of the juices. Flip the bread over and sprinkle the basil and cheese on top. Place under the grill to gently melt the cheese.

Cut the bread into little bite-sized pieces and serve warm.

Cheese and Chive
Stuffed Potatoes

Soft, fluffy mashed potato formed into little balls and stuffed with goat's cheese, then rolled in breadcrumbs and baked – a really tasty way to get your baby to eat mashed potato without the mess. These also work well as a side to Christmas dinner!

Serves 2 adults and 2 children

450g mashed potato

small bunch fresh chives, finely chopped

1 tablespoon parsley, finely chopped

2 tablespoons olive oil

1 teaspoon Dijon mustard

40g buffalo mozzarella, grated

1 egg, beaten

40g breadcrumbs

4 tablespoons rapeseed oil

Place the mashed potato in a bowl, add the chives, parsley, olive oil and mustard and mash until fluffy and soft.

Take a heaped tablespoon of mash in your hand and roll into a ball. Then take about half a teaspoon of mozzarella and press into the centre of the ball. Reshape, covering the mozzarella completely with the potato. Do this until all of the mash has been used up.

When you are finished, place the beaten egg in a bowl. Place the breadcrumbs in a separate bowl. Take each ball of potato and dip into the egg and then the breadcrumbs.

Heat the rapeseed oil in a frying pan. Then add the potato balls to the pan and cook until golden brown all over.

Serve warm.

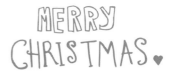

MERRY CHRISTMAS ♥

Index

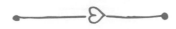